Praise for

Wow! *A Way Out* has forever changed my life and the way I view food and medicine. Matthew Grace is a genius and his book is full of insight and truth. Share this book with every one, it will change the world.

—Rory Freedman, Author of *Skinny Bitch*

Chapter 1 into this book, I was sold. This book lays out the TRUTH about everything food related and how it applies to the lives we live. He speaks on how things really are in the slaughterhouse. I found that chapter very disturbing, but it was good to know the truth. It made me forever look at cuts of meat in a different light.

As profound and insightful as this book was, with its hard hitting data and info, I still laughed aloud several times throughout the book. He's got a good sense of humor. All in all, top notch read for any vegetarian, or anyone wishing to improve their quality of life. His recovery from an incurable disease just puts the medical world to shame, and I love to see that. Instead of robbing people, let's help people.

—Mark T Brody

Mr. Grace's views needs to reach everyone. I will share this with everyone I care about, and how drastically it has changed my life in such a short amount of time. It doesn't have to be hard, people! We are the only ones that make it hard for ourselves. Live the way nature intended, and you will feel happier and more energetic, you will be in control of your body and emotions, and you'll never worry about disease again.

—Chastity Hope

This book changed my Life. Remember when the entire world believed the world was flat? Well, get ready—this book finally exposes the terrible myths of the "healthy" modern diet and opens your eyes to the truth of what we are actually eating. The key to REAL health is explained—backed by simple endless facts—a superb jolt to the old system of disease-causing diet beliefs. After reading this book, I'd be shocked if anyone could joyfully grab another bacon cheeseburger ever again! Seriously, read this book and decide for yourself! And by the way—I used LOVE cheeseburgers and I AM NEVER GOING BACK!!

I loved reading this book. It is well written with common sense that I believe can't be ignored. I recommend anyone read this book.

—Joy Kind

Matthew Grace has brought light into a world of darkness for anyone willing to follow his wisdom. I am grateful that he made it available for me in a time of need. It is a road map to read, study and absorb. YOU WILL benefit, I have. With much gratitude . . . thank you Matthew

—M Barlow

I found this book incredibly helpful in learning the truth about health and disease. My whole life, I loved dairy products, seafood, you name it. After reading this book, I went vegan—cutting out all animal products. Matthew Grace clearly demonstrated how most of our "health problems" are really side-effects of the way we eat. This book should be required reading for everyone, but especially people suffering from any diseases, and anyone interested in raw food diets.

—Nap nyc

From micro and macro viewpoints, Grace carefully dissects the 'myths' surrounding disease and contagion, from the black plaque in the Middle Ages to the modern plaques of obesity and cancers. It's fascinating and controversial stuff. Plus, there's a (often hilarious) take-down of the profit-hungry health care, dairy and beef industries, their mind-numbing propaganda, and the `hapless celebrities' that do their bidding. It's a page-turner—seriously! I didn't expect that from a book about health.

—C. Cooney

Matthew Grace's journey is an incredible testament to the healing powers of the body if you just give it the right tools.

—Chris Spartz

Matthew's words are so powerful because they blossomed from a lifetime of personal experience which has transformed into utmost passion and dedication to all those he encounters. He lives his life showing people what optimal health for the whole person looks and feels like; mind, body, spirit. His writing truly provides "A Way Out" from negative, limiting health beliefs, into positive beliefs about what it means to achieve a healthy life; not only for ourselves, but for our world.

—GABRIELLE ANGRESSANO

A Way Out is an outstanding book. In our economically driven society, we have gotten away from the truth about health. Matthew Grace reveals truth and common sense wisdom regarding nutrition and well being. He teaches us how to live according to the laws of nature. As a health professional, I give *A Way Out* my highest recommendation. Bravo!

— DR FEDELE E.VERO

Matthew Grace was crippled and diagnosed with "incurable disease." He refused all treatments and contrary to the allopathic prognoses, he worked himself back to superior health and strength. He is now a tireless and fierce advocate for proper nutrition and health. He has made himself onto a walking billboard for his methods and his book, *A Way Out* pulls no punches.

—HOWARD STRAUS, AUTHOR OF *HEALING THE HOPELESS*
AND HOST OF *THE POWER OF NATURAL HEALING*,
VOICEAMERICA HEALTH AND WELLNESS CHANNEL

Scientific and medical research has demonstrated that chronic diseases can be prevented by right dietary and lifestyle changes. Emerging cutting-edge research shows that our gut microbiome is instrumental in influencing every aspect of our mental and physical health; and the gut microbiome is in turn primarily influenced by diet. Matthew Grace in his book, *A Way Out*, indeed shows us a way out of dis-ease by presenting a life-enhancing, pragmatic, actionable, easy-to-implement plan on diet and lifestyle changes. This book in clear, lucid writing, filled with delicious recipes, is unputdownable and a must-read for anyone who strives to be their healthiest self to yield a life-long benefit!

—SHASHIREKHA MUNDHRA, PHD IMMUNOLOGY
AND MICROBIAL PATHOGENESIS

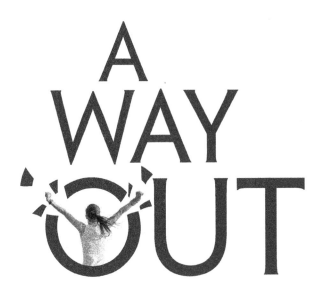

A WAY OUT

DISEASE DECEPTION & THE
TRUTH ABOUT HEALTH

MATTHEW GRACE

INFINITY LANE MEDIA

Published by Infinity Lane Media
www.matthewgrace.com

ISBN 978-1-7320623-0-6

Cover and chapter icon photo by
Shutterstock © lzf
Author photo by Andrew Brucker

Book design by DesignforBooks.com

DISCLAIMER
Matthew Grace is not a medical doctor and does
not prescribe medicine and or treatments for
disease. This book is a study of The Laws of Nature
and is an attempt to remind the reader that health
is a natural birthright, simple, and attainable by all.

DEDICATION

To all the great and brave souls
who have had the courage to tell the truth
in a world full of lies.

CONTENTS

*To Great Nature who never
stops teaching and reminding us
of the miraculous world in
which we live.*

INTRODUCTION

I magine being in a dark and crowded room. With every other step, you smash your shin on a table, hit your head on a lamp, smack your hip on the corner of a desk, and repeatedly trip over pieces of furniture. Everyone else is tripping and injuring him or herself also. You make efforts to stop injuring yourself, but despite your good intentions, you keep falling. There is somebody who is giving out pills that will deaden the pain of your injuries, and the pills are very popular in the land of the dark, as everybody is suffering cuts and bruises.

A collective decision is made to raise money in hopes of figuring out how to make furniture that is not so dangerous and to design clothing that will protect everyone from injury. The decision to name all the injuries suffered from particular falls and collisions is also agreed upon, including B.H.S. (Bruised Hip Syndrome), T.A. (Twisted Ankleitis), and B.H.D. (Bruised Head Disease). These acronyms are repeatedly used by physicians and the general population until they become part of the daily lexicon. Committees are formed, money is raised, celebrities (out of the goodness of their heart) speak out to increase "awareness." Research begins to find the "cures"

"The mind of man is taken far more with disguises than with realities"

≈ RALPH WALDO EMERSON

of these conditions. Experts suggest that walking faster will help, but more people end up getting injured. An expert from a top university claims it must be some type of microbe, either a germ or a virus, causing people to bang into furniture. Another expert says his study shows that walking backward is the answer, yet another claims the problem to be a genetic predisposition and begins lobbying for additional funds for genetic research. The years go on and on, and despite billions of dollars spent on this research and the advice of highly educated men and women, the people in the dark continue to trip and fall at an increasing rate. *Lack of money or lack of proper treatments and "cures" is not the issue.*

As long as you're in the dark it really does not matter what you decide, how intent you are at not banging into the furniture, how much research is done, or what the experts say.

The only *REAL* solution is to turn on the light.

Our civilization is the midst of a severe health crisis. Despite the fact that an entity called "Health Care" exists here in the United States, real health care does not exist. Disease management, precipitous, knee-jerk surgeries and drug sales are what passes for "Health Care." Health Education for the populace is as nonexistent as health education is for the doctors who oddly enough are in charge of our health. Those who are in charge of our health are failing miserably and we as a nation just keep getting sicker. Pharmaceutical companies continue to rake in billions and the populace just gets sicker. We are stumbling in the dark searching for solutions in places they simply do not exist. We live in a world where few, if any, human beings die of natural causes. To die of natural causes, you must live a natural life. In today's modern culture, people live unnatural lives and thus die of unnatural causes. Most human beings succumb to heart dis-ease and cancer treatments and die with debilitated and decrepit, disease-filled bodies, brittle and weakened bones, and failing organs. We are stumbling around in the dark imagining that if we run faster, raise more money, and do more research, things may improve. This is our present plight, but it does not have to be so.

The following work is offered as a safe and tremendously effective option for those who are suffering from dis-ease and physical discomfort, whether labeled incurable, chronic, or hereditary, and for those who simply want to live with optimum health.

My wish is that you read and re-read this book with *new ears*. It is not so much *IF* you read this book but how you read this book. Please do not fall into the trap of "I've already heard that," or "oh, that's just like what I learned at that seminar," etc. This is a horrible practice that disallows you to perceive what is really being said instead of your version or interpretation of what is being said. You may hear many words that you have heard before, but perhaps they may be saying something utterly different and altogether separate from what you may already know. Only an empty cup can be filled.

The general mass of our population is not exposed to the thousands of recoveries that take place every year from *all* types of dis-ease, whether deemed "incurable" or not. Those who *understand* the way the human body works and those who abide by these Laws of Nature invariably regain their health.

The aim of this work is to present you with knowledge that will enrich your life and present to you a path to health that *really* works. These principles are not my ideas, they are the impersonal, timeless, primordial and eternal Laws of Nature. Much like great scientists who have represented and reported their observations of the natural world, this work is an attempt to describe what has been observed in nature without the distorting and tainted effects of opinion (it has been said that opinion exists between ignorance and knowledge) or "beliefs of the day." Whether you are suffering from what is called chronic, incurable, or terminal dis-ease or you just want to lose weight, look better, or feel better, these laws will provide you with the best opportunity to do just that, simply, inexpensively and more effectively than anything else.

Years ago I was told that I had an *"incurable"* dis-ease. Wheelchair-bound, I was unable to move my legs, unable to stand or to walk, constantly fatigued, and suffering severe numbness throughout my body. I was told by doctors that I had no chance of recovery, and a couple of the doctors sympathetically encouraged me to enroll in a handicapped employment service. I was told of the list of steroids and other drugs given to those in my condition. The doctors could not tell me for sure what caused this dis-ease, how to cure it or say for certain if the drugs had any beneficial effect. Of course, all of the drugs prescribed had damaging effects, commonly called *"side"* effects. I therefore, refused ALL of their treatments, as none of them made any sense to me.

I am now back to a vigorous exercise regime that includes bicycle riding, yoga, rebounding (mini-trampoline), running, calisthenics, and, weight training.

For the past 30 years, I have witnessed the powerful and immutable Laws of Nature restore health to the sickest and seemingly hopelessly ill people, whether they were diagnosed with cancer, tumors, arthritis, chronic digestive problems, obesity, hypoglycemia, "aids," or diabetes. Those who commit themselves and adhere to nature's wisdom return themselves to health.

The idea that there is such a thing as "incurable dis-ease" is simply not true. Disease is just that . . . Dis-ease or lack of ease in the body.

Just as quickly as nature aids those who live in accordance with her laws, those who refuse to recognize these tenets suffer and are forced to exist in the confusion, darkness, and fear of our presently accepted notions of health and dis-ease, habitually resorting to dangerous and often deadly drugging and invasive surgeries. Nature is unforgiving. No matter how acceptable or revered our physicians and their treatments of the day may be, Natural Laws remain unaffected. *When you disregard Nature's Laws, it doesn't matter who is in agreement with you or what expert*

"The major cause of your illness: you have forgotten your true nature"

≡✲ BOETHIUS,
CONSOLATION OF PHILOSOPHY

advice you are following. You will pay the price. No one, no matter how educated or respected, can fly a lead kite.

The present paradigm for dealing with dis-ease is failing miserably, while nature's way continues to provide relief and healing to those who have sought out the truth and have been willing to make the necessary changes.

Our *"health experts"* provide us with drug after drug and treatment after treatment, yet the health of our citizens continues to decline. Despite billions of dollars spent on forty years of research and trillions of dollars on "treatments," more people today suffer from cancer than ever before, and still, no "cure" exists. At the same time, the cancer rate continues to climb. No real solutions have been found, just an ever-increasing number of treatments. Cancer screening tests are often free or extremely cheap. The *"treatments"* however, are a different story.

> *"Great truths do not take hold of the hearts of the masses."*
>
> ≋✿ CHUANG-TSE

Few, if any of us, understand doctors' methods of diagnosis and ask nothing about the remedies dispensed. Despite our confusion, we assume that what we are being told is the truth and the most effective course of action in the treatment of our symptoms.

There are countless *"health experts"* on the scene with new protocols and treatments for the sick, all professing that they have the answer to treating dis-ease. Year after year, new and exciting (often bizarre) techniques are introduced to an ignorant public who is promised *"miracle cures"* and *"wonder drugs."* Watch a newscast this evening, and you have a good chance to hear about a *"hopeful"* new drug or medical *"breakthrough."*

Despite the continuous hype, nobody seems to recognize the emptiness of these promises or the continuing decline of our health. The confusion deepens with each passing fad and mania. True health remains a mystery to the masses.

Why is it that health has become such a confusing issue? Has the creative force that put together this amazing universe made a mistake? Why is it that animals (in their pristine environment) do not live such dis-eased lives? There are no epidemics in the pristine natural world. Outbreaks of arthritis, asthma, cancer, obesity, heart dis-ease, strokes, "aids," osteoporosis, flu's etc., do not exist in the untainted natural world. No animals in nature are injecting themselves with dangerous vaccines or flu shots. There are no animals taking supplements or protein powders or going on diets, eating according to their blood type, or eating "like cavemen," or weighing their food. They simply abide by their natural instincts and get along just fine.

Unfortunately, our natural instincts concerning nutrition are buried DEEP beneath the morass of misinformation and propaganda that exists in today's world. We are submerged in a sea of illusions and deceptions that are so rampant and persuasive that the truth is virtually out of our realm of consideration. The power of our natural intuition has been all but nullified by our "schooling" and the ubiquitous presence of big business. The medical lobby in Washington is second only to the oil lobby in its influence on lawmakers.

Oil companies and drug companies have a long, intertwined and sordid history. The pharmaceutical business itself actually began with John Rockefeller selling off the by-product of his refined oil as an elixir for cancer and constipation. He called it "Nujol" and bottled it for 1/5th of a penny and sold it for twenty-six cents a bottle. A staggering profit, and there began the pharmaceutical industry. Nujol caused great health hazards as it robbed the body of fat-soluble vitamins. That did not stop Senator Royal S. Copeland, former health commissioner of New York City, from taking $75,000.00 a year from Mr. Rockefeller (equal to 1.3 Million dollars per year in today's world) to promote Nujol on the radio health show he broadcast from the US Senate building every morning. Today you will be hard pressed to find ANY pharmaceuticals that do not have petrochemicals included.

As an interesting side note, Rockefeller refused to take ANY drugs and had a Homeopath for his private doctor. His name was Harrold Biggar.

Modern medicine's deluded misrepresentations concerning health and dis-ease have so heavily indoctrinated our day-to-day thinking that an outside, objective observer would see little chance for most people to think clearly about these issues. The mental corruption runs so deep that there are only a small number of citizens that are even willing to listen to another point of view.

Our unconscious acceptance of such specious and misleading information from our "experts" is the reason why we are at the mercy of dis-ease and powerless to question our doctors and their diagnosis of our illnesses and choice of treatments.

Are human bodies flawed?

Is there any reason why dis-ease has become a part of our everyday life and accepted as natural? Did nature make some mistakes when designing the human body? Why are we the only species on the planet that suffer such dis-ease ridden lives? Alas, we are NOT the only species on the planet that suffer disease. Our house pets also become obese, get arthritis, suffer toothaches, have upset stomachs, experience cancer and the rest of the gamut of pain that humans endure. What is the common denominator between our house-pets and ourselves?

The glaring and most obvious factor is the quality of food that we and our house-pets ingest. This food is of a completely different quality than what is ingested in nature.

We are the only species on the planet eating cooked, devitalized food.

Nature has provided EVERYTHING necessary for life; Sunshine, air, water and the necessary instincts to stay out of harm's way. Nature has not forgotten anything. The complete recipe for our well-being and dis-ease free lives is at hand. The question must be asked. Why is it that we suffer so much dis-ease?

Pain is the great messenger.

Pain is always trying to get a message to us. It is an indication that something is amiss, and an adjustment must be made to return our selves back to comfort. If the actions taken to remove the pain do not work or, worse, exacerbate the pain, it ought to be an indication that our efforts need to be re-examined. Our modern civilization is in a lot of pain. The methods presently practiced are increasing our pain, as more people are suffering dis-ease than ever before. If we were truly serious about solving this problem, the answers could be found.

However, a major problem exists in our society. We are tuned in to the QUICK FIX mentality. We have a headache, and we want immediate relief and so reach for a pain-killer or an aspirin. Our stomach is upset, so we take something to quell the symptom for instant relief. We are feeling empty so we overeat . . . very rarely do we consider the message that is being sent to us by our bodies or spend a minute wondering about the possible CAUSE of our discomfort. Instead, we create a pattern of numbing and suppressing the body which, in turn, creates a veritable gagging of nature's communication with us. This impatient, automatic reaction to obtain relief is a major cause of our dire health crises.

If your wish for relief is greater than your wish for understanding, you will get neither genuine relief, nor genuine understanding.

Imagine a dammed lake that is being continuously flooded by an over-flowing river. The added pressure creates cracks in the wall of the dam. A messenger boy repeatedly rides into town to tell the leaders of the village that there are cracks in the dam. Instead of gathering some engineers and going to see for themselves in order to assess the damage and pinpoint the cause of the cracks, the town leaders give the young boy some plaster and spackling tools and tell him to keep quiet about the news of the weakening dam so as not to upset the townspeople. The leaders, convinced by each other that they have done the right thing, go on about their business disregarding the imminent warnings. The young boy is able to do some temporary repairs. Cosmetically, the dam appears fine, but appearances cannot fool the Laws of Nature . . . disaster is imminent.

This is an example of foolish decision makers disregarding signs of impending doom. Though deep down they sense the wrongness of it, they convince each other that sending the messenger boy to mend the cracks in the wall is a responsible and appropriate measure. Their nodding heads and collective agreements may provide a temporary and false feeling of comfort, but this charade will not affect the inevitable outcome.

Modern society does the same when dealing with disease. When any physical discomfort or distress appears, we take a pill to alleviate the pain; this quick and cosmetic approach *does nothing to remove the CAUSE of the pain.* This is today's accepted and "normal" method of dealing with pain or discomfort yet it is no different than the ignorant and dangerous act of silencing the messenger boy and sending him to spackle the wall of a collapsing dam.

Not only does this method of suppressing symptoms negate the need for any understanding of the cause of pain, the substances that are used to mask the pain can cause many more bodily sufferings to come.

Quick-fix solutions lead to long-term disasters.

The insanity of this covering up and disregarding the body's message is dangerous enough, but if one takes the time to consider the very substances used for the masking, with all their inherent deleterious, dis-ease producing effects, the madness of the whole process begins to reveal itself.

ALL drugs and pharmaceutical products have what the doctors and drug companies call "side" effects, which are debilitating symptoms caused by the very substance that is supposed to be making us well. These "side" effects may include everything from headaches, vomiting, and fevers to kidney failure, heart failure, and that annoying little "SIDE" effect known as death. Indeed, there are actually drugs that list death as a possible "side effect."

In other words, if a healthy person were to take ANY drug, they would be made ill.

Does it make any sense to give a sick person a drug that will make a healthy person sick in order to make a sick person healthy?

Let us be very clear about one thing: *There is no such thing as "side" effects. These effects are direct and frontal assaults on your health.* Many times these side effects are worse than the original symptoms, and many symptoms known as "latter stages" of dis-ease (cancer, "aids" and diabetes, etc.) are in fact caused by these toxic and often lethal treatments. It is very rare that a patient dies of cancer, despite what we are told. Most patients diagnosed with cancer die from the side effects of their highly toxic chemo-"therapy." Through the guise of "early detection saves lives" and fear-inducing admonitions by doctors and ignorant celebrities, more people than ever are being diagnosed and "treated" for cancer. Only in a very confused world would people subject themselves to having mustard gas injected into their veins, having breasts removed as a "preventative" measure, and succumbing to radiation "treatments" in hopes of becoming healthy, not to mention paying inordinate sums of money for these procedures. The death rate from cancer (and cancer "treatments") continues to climb.

Our present and accepted methods of "healthcare" are insane. In fact, *there is no such thing as true health care in modern medicine.* There is only dis-ease classification, disease management, and drug salesmanship. Doctors, in their myopic approach to dis-ease, are blind to the ways of health, and hospitals lack EVERY essential for our well-being. Without sunshine or fresh air, hospitals offer toxic dis-ease producing foods and drinks, daily druggings and "treatments" and an atmosphere of patient powerlessness. A "good" (meaning obedient) patient has much less of a chance to get out alive or unscathed as a patient with a mind of his or her own.

Doctors are Unschooled in Health

I am first in line to applaud and admire the medical techniques, procedures, and skills of the doctors that mend broken bones, damaged tendons, and torn cartilage. Their skills and artistry in this area of reconstruction and structural repair are a tremendous boon to our civilization, allowing people to live their lives with greater comfort and ability. However, as far as their perspective and treatment of dis-ease go, there is little to admire.

Doctors study dis-ease (health failure) and drug use. Because of the constant influx of new drugs that don't work, to replace the old ones that do not work, their "education" depends on the drug salesmen who represent the very companies that profit from the doctors' prescriptions. It is common practice for salesmen to give away free samples and offer perks such as free vacations, cash, and other gifts to doctors if they can sell a certain amount of a new product. Drug companies will pay in full for luxurious vacations at the finest resorts and will invite scores of doctors and hospital administrators in order to "*educate*" them on the benefits of their new products.

The following is a list of direct quotes from a man who practiced medicine for over thirty years. He is no longer with us, but his words are as valuable as ever to those who are committed to regaining their health and protecting their families and loved ones.

"Whenever you are in a hospital, you are in mortal danger."

"One of the unwritten rules of modern medicine is always to write a prescription for new drugs quickly before side effects have come to the surface."

"Doctors are not trained to attack the core of any problem, merely to suppress the symptoms."

"Doctors should be treated with about the same amount of trust as used car salesmen."

"I believe that more than ninety percent of modern medicine could disappear from the face of the earth—doctors hospitals, drugs, and equipment—and the effect on our health would be immediate and beneficial."

—Dr. Robert Mendelsohn, *Confessions of a Medical Heretic*

Dr. Mendelsohn was an associate professor at the University of Illinois Medical School and the director of Chicago's Michael Reese Hospital. He wrote a syndicated column called *The People's Doctor* and was chairman of the Medical Licensure Committee for the state of Illinois. This man was educated by and worked in the heart of the medical establishment. His efforts to report what other doctors deny and keep secret are a testament to his courage and veracity. He was a heroic man with a sense of decency who truly-honored his physician's creed FIRST DO NO HARM. There are so few doctors who are willing to tell the truth about their profession (and apparently so few patients that ever question them) because the doctors who do inevitably suffer persecution and vilification from the AMA and mainstream society. These are some of the doctors who have stood up for

"Doctors pour drugs of which they know little—to cure diseases of which they know less—into human beings of which they know nothing."

≋ VOLTAIRE

truth and the healing powers of Nature's Laws, despite the grave consequences and denigration they undoubtedly endured:

Dr. John Tilden	Dr. William Alcott
Dr. Russell Trail	Dr. Nicholas Gonzalez
Dr. Sylvester Graham	Dr. T.V. Gifford
Dr. Issac Jennings	Dr. Joseph Mercola
Dr. Susanna W. Dodds	Dr. Robert Willner

There are a few doctors who presently are willing to be truthful about all they do not know and the dangerous practices of modern medicine, and they are vigorously persecuted for their honesty.

Our mechanical reaction to seek out a doctor for health advice needs, to be fully examined if we are serious about our well being.

"There are more things in heaven and earth than are dreamt of in your philosophies."

≋ SHAKESPEARE

Let us say you wanted to learn how to sing. Would you seek out an auto mechanic to teach you? Of course not. That is an absurd idea, as auto mechanics (as a rule) are not schooled in the art of voice and would be unable to help you attain the necessary skills. You would seek out somebody who is an expert vocalist. *If health is what you want, why would you go to somebody who studies the failure of health (disease)?* If you wanted to become a millionaire would you go to skid row to interview the homeless and destitute about their financial planning skills?

If you are interested in health, it would make sense to STUDY HEALTH. The problem is that our perception of what health is remains quite distorted, and the possibility exists that we really do not have a human model for health. Certainly, modern medicine's use of a "normal" man or woman (feeding on unnatural foods and poisoning themselves forty to fifty times a day) as a model for health is baseless and absurd.

The intention of this work is to provide the reader with a sane and logical guideline to health. The problems that exist concerning health are listed as well as the solutions.

The program is simple yet quite challenging to those of the civilized, fast food, quick-fix world, but it is *unimaginably rewarding*. It is also cheap, convenient and wonderfully effective, see for yourself.

There is also no pressure to do this immediately or completely. You might want to make some diligent efforts to incorporate some of these principles and see for yourself if your health and vitality does not improve.

I remember the days when I first came across this knowledge of natural feeding and thought how sensible and logical it sounded despite the fact that I was eating close to the standard, American (or S.A.D.) diet. I thought how difficult it was going to be to give up my favorite foods—i.e. pizza, cheeseburgers, ice cream, etc.

Yes, I can honestly tell you that the very foods I dreaded giving up are presently completely unappealing to me, and many of them seem downright disgusting. I am in disbelief about many of the things I used to eat on a daily basis. Certainly, if somebody told me, thirty-five years ago that I would be a raw-foodist and no longer eat the foods I was so completely attached to and be completely content, I would have told them that they were nuts. I had no reference at that time for this way of living and all its life-enhancing, exquisite benefits. You may be in the same situation. Give this program a try . . . you can always go back to your former ways.

There was a friend of mine who would periodically talk to me about the harmful effects of animal products, and I responded with impatience, disrespect, and often light-hearted ridicule about the one or two vegetarians I knew. This was my short-sighted, uninformed impression of the knowledge that was being offered to me, and I wanted no part of it. As my willingness to hear the truth increased, so did my health and happiness.

It is very difficult for us to hear information that challenges our comfort zones and settled ideas. However, making these kinds of efforts is SO essential to our overall growth as human beings, and so tremendously exciting with results that are almost immediately measurable. It is a wonderful thing to UNDERSTAND health and live according to the Laws of Nature. To eat with consciousness and no longer add to the suffering that is so rampant on our planet, to no longer partake of foods that are destroying our ecology and our health, and to no longer feel at the mercy of dis-ease or fear old age and the onset of a debilitated body. What a gift it is to find a lifestyle that provides one with autonomy over one's health.

If you or a loved one have been told that you are doomed to live with "incurable" or "chronic" dis-ease, you have been lied to. You do not have to suffer through the druggings, burnings, poisonings, mutilations, irradiations, and hopelessness prescribed to you. You now have the opportunity to do what thousands of others have done. You can take responsibility for your well being and understand the true nature of dis-ease and the simplicity of health and allow your body to do what it knows best—heal.

Remember, Health is our natural state.

There is one disease on the planet and one cure

The disease is toxicity, and the cure is detoxification.

Detoxifying the body from physical poisons is a great start and maybe all you need to do to get well. You may also need to rid yourself of toxic thoughts and emotions as well . . . Not necessarily in that order.

Any disease from cancer to diabetes, to asthma, to a cold, to the flu, etc., has to do with the body's response to physical and or emotional poisoning. The average American poisons themselves (physically) an average of fifty times a day. There is no telling how many times we poison ourselves with our thinking and our emotions. When the poisoning ceases, health begins to return.

Naming your disease and saying "I have _____" is not going to help you. Stating what you wish for yourself will help you. Don't use the name modern medicine gives to your list of symptoms, it will not help you. Instead, state what you wish for yourself. "I am becoming a strong healthy, fit person." Tell those around you as well to NOT use the medical terminology that only brings despair and hopelessness.

Don't believe what your doctor tells you concerning your chances of recovery. They do not know your possibilities.

In this edition of A WAY OUT I have added a few extra chapters. Pay close attention to Giving Birth and Raising Your Healthy Child (chapter 10). This chapter is filled with a large amount of vital content that will do nothing but aid you on your path to Health. Even if you do not plan on having a child it is well worth reading.

1

THE DISASTER OF
ANIMAL PRODUCTS

For the first twenty years of my life, I was raised on the standard American diet (S.A.D.), and I rarely, if ever, questioned the idea of what I was ingesting. I loved bacon, cheeseburgers, ham, steak, and all the "normal" foods that our society accepts. I also believed these foods were necessary for my health and well being. It is a common belief that eating animal products is essential for building muscle and keeping our strength up. As an athlete, I certainly did not want to jeopardize my strength or ability to build muscle, and I did not begin to seriously question what I ate until the age of twenty-one.

Being a meat-eater for so long a period of time makes it difficult to judge anybody for the unconscious eating habits that I, myself, practiced for years. This information had not found me yet, and, in my ignorance, there was no problem with the way I was living my life, blind to

"It is 'my view that the vegetarian manner of living, by its purely physical effect on the human temperament, would most beneficially influence the lot of mankind.'

≅✴ ALBERT EINSTEIN

the truth of what eating animals entailed and all its catastrophic consequences. I was completely trusting of what I had been told, I did as others did. Having knowledge of the information that follows made it impossible for me to continue on, thankfully so. Leaving off the eating of animals has deepened my compassion for ALL life on Earth and has made a huge impact on the quality of my health.

Certainly, the following chapter may be disturbing, and there is no doubt that many people do not want to read about the accepted mayhem and brutality our society condones and supports. It was not very popular to be one of the first abolitionists, as slavery was acceptable and rarely questioned by the masses. According to many, even "men of God," certain colored men were supposed to own different colored men. If you were a woman and wanted to vote one hundred years ago, most people would think that you were a "radical" or a "revolutionist," as the idea of a woman voting was offensive. These were the time-honored, conventional practices of the day and were not to be questioned.

Is there any doubt that those who were brave enough to originally express their opposition to these perverse practices were scoffed at and ridiculed for their conscientious opposition? Will there come a time when the present-day heinous disregard and brutal treatment of animals are viewed with the same indignation and disgust we have today towards slavery and discrimination?

The following pages, which focus on the treacherous effects of our animal-based diet, are written with the intention of shining light on all that has been in the dark and hidden from mainstream society for so many years. It is shocking information. Shocks are often necessary to awaken a sleeping public.

The films our country saw of the Vietnam war completely changed the way we view war. Because of the daily documentation of the atrocities of this particular war, the reality of war itself was made real in the minds of our citizens. It was no longer some type of innocuous John Wayne movie where the good guys beat the bad guys. The pictures told the real and graphic story of the insane hell that war is. Because of this shock, public outcry against the war increased, and the war was mercifully ended years before it might have been without that revealing media exposure.

There is an equally atrocious, vile, and violent set of circumstances that exist today, the scope of which has yet to be realized by the general population. For whatever reasons, these events have gone unnoticed and have remained hidden from the mainstream. We are all doing the best we can with what we know, and I believe that our existence here on Earth would change dramatically if we were more informed.

Please read the following with an open and objective mind and see if it makes sense to you. It may be uncomfortable to read and against your intellectual and emotional attachments, but remember that all improvements (of yourself and the world) require significant and consistent effort and a certain degree of discomfort. These noble efforts that go against our comfort zones and heighten our consciousness are the very struggles that advance us as individuals and as a people and, as such, are the only genuinely lasting rewards of life on Earth.

Protein

"Where do you get your protein?" This most commonly asked question to those who leave off the eating of animals and eat according to the Laws of Nature is best answered by a series of other questions: Where does a horse get its protein? Where does an ox get its protein? Where does a rhinoceros or an elephant get its protein? All of these incredibly muscular and powerful animals are herbivores that eat nothing but plant life yet, they have immense strength and vitality.

Folklore teaches us that the Lion is the "king of the jungle," That idea is a joke. As a single lion would never attack a full grown elephant, water buffalo or rhinoceros as these animals would badly injure and/or kill ANY lion that tried to do so. Lions hunt in packs and they always pick the slowest and weakest prey to attack. Not so noble or regal is the lion.

It is true that these animals have a physiology that is quite different from that of a human being. However one of the strongest mammals on the planet is the silverback gorilla who has an almost identical digestive system to ours, and the many physiological similarities between our two species are quite evident. Despite being anywhere from two to three times as large as a human being, these gorillas are TEN times as strong. These animals have an incredibly powerful physique and ingest nothing but plant life.

How is it and why is it that our society is so convinced that we need to ingest a large amount of protein and animal products to be strong and healthy while the example nature sets go unnoticed? We eat the flesh of a cow for the protein, yet all the cow eats in its natural environment is the grass. If all the aforementioned animals feed themselves exclusively with plant life, why is it that we are so concerned with "getting enough protein?"

Have you ever heard of anybody with a protein deficiency?

The protein myth has been developed, like all myths, by people repeating things they have been told instead of verifying those ideas as factual for themselves.

Repeat a lie long enough and loud enough and it becomes a "reality."

This is an old and reliable recipe for brainwashing the masses. "Realities" are formed by collective agreement and often have nothing to do with the truth.

We do not have to think too far back to remember the days of the oft-mentioned "four food groups," two of which were "meat and dairy" products. One would be hard-pressed to find one of these pamphlets or food charts that was not put together by the meat industry or the dairy council. As far as the "reality" of the four food groups goes, there is absolutely NO scientific, physiological or biological evidence to support this recommended nutritional guideline that our doctors and physicians embarrassingly promulgated for more than thirty years. This salesmanship by certain businesses and backed by "health professionals" has caused untold numbers of diseased, dying, and dead citizens.

Mercifully, the four food groups fiasco has ended, yet the myth of getting enough protein continues to grow and hover in the unconscious belief system of the masses. It is a wonderful marketing ploy to scare the unknowing public into believing that they need to have a certain food product or their health will deteriorate. It is especially effective when "experts" repeat the lies in order to sell specious products, much the same way doctors used to recommend and advertise cigarettes to the television audiences of the fifties and sixties, obviously helping to increase the possibility of lung cancer and death in exchange for a few bucks from the tobacco companies.

Scientifically speaking, the definition of a protein is a chain link of amino acids. In other words . . .

Amino acids are the building blocks of protein.

According to our scientists, there are twenty-three different types of amino acids, eight of which they claim are "essential." They are ALL essential. According to our present scientists, the body produces fifteen amino acids, and the other eight must be derived from our food intake. If you are eating even a small array of fruits, you are receiving every amino acid and nutrient you need, just as animals in nature are well nourished as they abide by their instincts.

There is no greater source, in terms of both quantity and quality, for amino acids than raw fruits, raw vegetables, raw seeds and nuts. These are the same fruits and vegetables our plant-eating animal friends in their natural environment use to build their amazing bodies and strength. There are no supplements or protein powders, and no animals weigh their food or add up their protein/carbohydrate intake and no animals eat according to their blood type. Are the power, vitality, and health of these species proof enough that nature has provided all the nutrients we need with plant food? Perhaps this evidence is logical and sensible to those who can TRULY think for themselves, an almost impossible task in our well-programmed society.

The most perfect human food on the planet, mother's milk, has only three percent protein. This food, designed by the supreme creator, is the food infants can eat exclusively to grow their bodies in the first years of life on Earth. It is a complete and perfect food, providing the mother is in good health, and is a clear indication that protein is not the most important nutrient for a human being.

Flesh foods provide no fuel or energy. In fact, despite the often stimulating effects of meat, it is incredibly devitalizing and enervating to the human body. It

takes tremendous energy to digest flesh foods. One of
the natural byproducts of cooked animal flesh digestion
is ammonia. The amino acids that carnivorous animals
use to build their bodies (while eating the meat raw of
course) are coagulated and destroyed through the process
of cooking. Not only is meat a poor source of protein,
it is toxic to the body and is dis-ease producing. Even
the AMA has documented cancer-causing effects of
ingesting cooked animal flesh. *The Journal of the National
Cancer Institute* says "heart dis-ease deaths and bowel
cancer deaths are directly proportional to meat consumption." The National Cancer Research Institute found that
women who eat daily portions of meat are four times
more likely to get breast cancer than those women who
eat little or no meat.

Animal products are *THE* prime source of the cholesterol that clogs arteries.

If it were recognized, this is a fact that could immediately
cut in half the number of those suffering from heart dis-
ease. Of course, the elimination of polyunsaturated fat and
hydrogenated oils found in margarine and other "low fat"
highly processed foods, along with the cessation of ingesting
animal products, would END the epidemic of arteriosclero-
sis, stroke, and heart attack from which we suffer.

Evidence of the benefits of a vegetarian diet has been
well documented. The healthiest people in the world,
the Hunzukuts, (or Hunzas) commonly live past the age
of one hundred, stay extremely active their entire lives,

and rarely experience any dis-ease. There are no pharmaceutical drugs, no formula drinks, no steroids, and no
osteoporosis. These people have been examined by western doctors such as Dr. Alexander Leaf who did a study
for National Geographic on the oldest people in the
world and the illustrious and prominent physician Dr.
Paul Dudley White who tendered President Eisenhower.
Besides finding no obesity, no cancer, and no diabetes,
they found NO HEART DISEASE. Dr. White did
a study on twenty-five men over the age of ninety and
found them to be, in perfect health. The Hunzas diet is
strictly vegetarian and eighty percent RAW FOOD. The
China Study written by T. Collin Campbell shows quite
clearly the benefits of a plant-based diet.

The Pythagoreans, Buddhists, Taoists and the
Essenes all regarded a vegetarian diet as a necessary discipline. In fact, according to many Biblical scholars such
as Ernest Renan (*Life of Jesus*), Jesus Christ himself was
an Essene and a vegetarian. From the Essene *Gospel of
Peace*, Christ is quoted: "Eat nothing to which the fire of
death gives savor, for such is Satan."

Many people will say "human beings have been eating
meat for thousands of years." Maybe that's true, maybe
not, as some anthropologists claim that the first human
beings were exclusively fruit eaters. The argument could
be made that we have also been murdering and torturing each other as well as waging wars for thousands of
years, right up to and through the present day "civilized"
world. These are practices that need to be examined. Just
because we've been doing something for a long time does
not mean it should not be questioned.

Let us take an objective look at this practice of killing and eating animals.

Physiologically speaking, there are clear and inarguable differences between the physical makeup of a carnivore and a human being. The first is the obvious lack of foot speed we have compared to flesh-eating animals. Every flesh eater is equipped with great speed and/or blinding quickness. The fastest human being in the world is nowhere near as fast as wild cats or dogs.

All carnivores' jaws are extremely powerful and move exclusively up and down which is extremely effective for ripping and tearing flesh. Plant eaters have jaws that move not only up and down but from side to side. This functional difference is plain to see in the animal kingdom.

Carnivores have fangs and claws effectively designed to inflict fatal wounds on their prey. We do not. Could you imagine trying to kill an animal without a gun, a knife, or some other type of weapon? Many carnivores have the strength and ability to bring down animals that are two to three times their size and weight. Their ability to kill is built-in, they need nothing other than that with which they were born. We cannot say that about our physiology. Imagine yourself confronting a full-sized deer, antelope, elephant, or giraffe with the intent to inflict a fatal blow. It would be a more than comical sight as well as quite dangerous to your well being. The animal might be somewhat confused at the sight of this harmless creature (you) standing before him with bad intentions but obviously ill-equipped to murder or even do any significant physical harm. Our physical strength is no match when compared to wild carnivorous animals.

There are those that claim that we have two "canine" teeth and argue that this is evidence that we were meant to eat meat. Let these people try to eat a raw piece of meat without the use of sharp knives, meat grinders, or food, processors. Then we can discuss their findings. Our teeth and jaws are set up for the chewing and mastication of plant life.

Our saliva is alkaline, carnivores have acid saliva. Carnivores' stomachs secrete ten times the amount of hydrochloric acid than human beings do. Hydrochloric acid is the vital and necessary substance used for flesh digestion. Our digestive systems are completely different. Further, carnivores have rough abrasive tongues, ours are smooth.

Millions of Americans and citizens of other "civilized" countries suffer from the painful, debilitating condition known as arthritis. When an animal is slaughtered all eliminative processes end at once, and the urine or uric acid that was marked for elimination remains in the flesh of the animal. Carnivores are equipped to deal with this ingested urine. They have an enzyme called uricase specifically designed for this purpose. Human beings do not have uricase. The massive amount of urine ingested by meat-eating humans beings is extremely difficult to process by our digestive system. After years of this filthy, unnatural habit of ingesting the dead, the uric acid begins to crystallize in a human body and is deposited in the joints causing the painful twisting and turning of the bones, stiffness, and lameness.

Doctors claim this condition to be "incurable." I have seen this condition repeatedly reversed and eliminated by those who end their carnivorous habits.

The intestines of a carnivorous animal are extremely short, only about three times the length of its body so that the unused ingested flesh food is dispelled quickly and the decaying flesh does not linger in the digestive tract of the animal. Human beings have intestines that reach twelve times the length of their trunk to allow for proper absorption of the needed nutrients derived from the ingested plant life. Flesh food in our digestive tract is a disaster, incredibly difficult and sometimes impossible to digest. Surgeons have reported on undigested flesh foods that do not break down and will remain stuck or impacted in a patient's digestive tract for YEARS.

It is common for lions and tigers to sleep twenty hours after feeding on flesh, an indication of the nerve energy used to break down their meal. It is also interesting to note that these carnivores do not eat other carnivores, and the first part of the vegetarian animal they eat is the intestines where all the water-rich plant life digests.

Psychological aspects of flesh-eating

Please give some serious thought to the following questions:

- What is your first reaction to seeing a dead animal?
- Are you interested?
- Do you have an impulse to get closer?
- Do you want to smell the stinking carcass?
- Do you want to taste it?

- ᴥ When you see some road kill, does it make you drool?
- ᴥ Does the sight or smell of a dead animal increase or decrease your appetite?
- ᴥ Is it accurate to say that your first reaction to a bloodied dead animal is revulsion?

The answers to these questions are obvious. Human beings are disgusted and repelled by the sight of dead, bloodied animals. As soon as the life force is ended, a body immediately begins to decompose and rot, causing a foul stench and an ugly sight, which is not very appetizing. Sure enough, this sight creates disgust and a natural instinct to stay away, this is hard to deny. Strangely enough, these rotting decaying cadavers have become the main "food" in our civilized society's diet. WHY? How could this be if our natural instinct towards a rotting cadaver is utter disgust? The natural instinct of our cats and dogs IS to sniff it and inspect it, however, most wild cats and dogs will not eat a carcass unless it has just been killed. Somehow eating "aged" meat has become some kind of a "delicacy" for our "civilized society." Only nature's scavengers, including vultures, hyenas, flies, worms, etc., will indulge in a rotting corpse. Human beings are not meant to be scavengers, and it is a blow to our dignity to partake in this filthy food and act as scavengers. "Don't touch it!" is what we yell at our children when coming across an animal corpse, then we walk to the picnic table and give them a corpse sandwich . . . to eat.

Perhaps it's a little unnerving or even shocking to refer to a hamburger or turkey sandwich as a "corpse" sandwich, yet that's exactly what it is. An apple is an apple, an orange is an orange, and a rotting decaying piece of flesh is a corpse. Eating a corpse is a ghoulish act. Of course, we are not inclined to think in this manner and have invoked many wonderful euphemisms for these animal cadavers. These linguistic niceties provide us with buffers and distract us from paying attention to just what it is that we eat on a daily basis. We do not eat sliced cadavers, we eat "cold cuts" or "hot dogs" or "hamburgers."

Confucius once said, when being asked how to uplift a fallen society, that the first order of business is to "rectify the language." This wise man understood that language can be used to control the populace and make them do things that are disastrous to their well being. Language plays a huge role in hypnotizing the masses. For instance, in this country, we have a "Defense" Department . . . that wages war. It used to be called the War Department. The "Defense" Department now refers to the battlefield as the "theater," kills as "casualties," and wars as "conflicts." We have a "healthcare" system in charge of dis-ease management that knows nothing about health, and "side" effects that kill you. George Orwell in his novel *1984* predicted that by the end of the twentieth-century language would be used as such a successful weapon against the people ("newspeak") that free speech and freedom of choice would not be possible.

The people who sell dead animals for food, along with our entire society, have agreed to an ingenious and impressive array of euphemisms to deal with the common practice of feeding on the dead. There are few people who would return to a restaurant if a steak were listed on the menu as "Dead Cow" or "Rotting Cadaver." That would not be polite. When selling treacherous products it is not good business to be candid or direct. So we are in the habit of invoking the romantic languages of France and Italy and other countries to eat and sell cadavers as food: "Filet mignon," "Chateaubriand," "Foie gras," (fat liver) "Veal scaloppini," "Filet of sole," "Steak tartar," "escargot" (snails). Most people would not eat snails on a dare, let alone pay thirty or forty bucks for this "delicacy," unless it carried with it the pretentious air of "sophistication" that it does. Next time you are in a restaurant, it might be interesting to order your food using simple and plain language: "I'll have the dead baby cow and the liver of a tortured goose with a glass of spoiled (fermented) red grape juice." Your waiter might give you a strange look, your friends could be disgusted, and you also might end up ordering a salad. Everyone would profit.

> *"You have just dined; and however scrupulously the slaughterhouse is concealed in the graceful distance of miles, there is complicity."*
> ➳ EMERSON

I wonder how many people would be able to go out and hack to death a docile, peaceful cow, sift through the gallons of blood and guts, and tear away some flesh to put upon the stove every time they wanted a hamburger, a roast beef sandwich, a hot-dog, or a steak?

If we were obliged to kill every time we wanted a piece of meat how would that affect the dietary habits of our culture?

What if our children understood that hamburgers do not

"grow in patches" as McDonalds will have them believe? What if they knew the fright and sheer terror these animals experienced before their violent execution? What if they knew the rush of adrenalin and fear that courses through the blood of these beings before they are slaughtered and that the hamburgers they eat are filled with that adrenaline and fear? What if they knew that these animals' were tortured their entire lives and suffered a horrific execution, being hung upside down by one leg (which immediately dislocates and often breaks) and had their throats cut until they bled to death? Maybe they would understand that becoming an Oscar Meyer Weiner (as the song goes) is not what they would wish for after all. Maybe they would not want to order their "Happy Meals" with such frequency. Maybe they would see that they are in fact Horror Meals and be rightfully afraid and unwilling to partake in such fiercely inhumane and brutally slaughtered gore.

> *"The time will come when men such as I will look on the murder of animals as they now look on the murder of men."*
> ≡✶ LEONARDO DA VINCI

The fact is that not just our children, but our entire population are carefully and intentionally kept very far away from the harsh, nightmarish brutality that goes on every day in this country. *There are ten million animals a day put to death in this country alone.* Despite that staggering number of killings, not many of us have ever seen what goes on in a slaughterhouse. Why is it that we are so far removed from these places of death if flesh eating is such a major and completely accepted part of our lives?

The answer is simple: It would be too horrible a sight and sound for most of our population to bear.

Animals can hear the screams, smell the stench, and often see the cows being put to death before them. Dr. Temple Grandin reports numerous cases of "deliberate cruelty" from the workers who "enjoy killing and tormenting animals on purpose," taking "sadistic pleasure from shooting the eyes out of cattle, striking them in the head, and electrically shocking them in sensitive areas of their bodies."

Before their throats are cut, these animals are hit with a pistol bolt set against each animal's head, and the metal rod is mechanically shot into the brain. Because the animal is often upset and fighting for its life, the bolt misses its mark creating tremendous pain:

> I saw with my own eyes innocent animals having their heads bashed in with a captive bolt pistol, some two or three times. Then a man would walk over and slit the cow's throat. Buckets of blood poured out. It was horrible—the animals were squirming and screaming. One of the men came out of a room while sharpening a knife and told us to watch out for cows who fall off the chain and charge the workers.
>
> —Mike Lace, Grant City, Illinois, April 1997

> A meat packing plant is like nothing you have ever seen or could imagine. It's like a vision of hell.
>
> —Eleanor Kennelly, United Food & Commercial Workers Union

It is an uplifting thing to have seen so many people *go* out of their way to take in abused and abandoned animals and compassionately take the time and spend the money to find loving homes for these unfortunate dogs and cats; yet it is an incongruous, bizarre event to see these very people eat a hot dog or hamburger without even a thought of the life of violence and abuse a cow or pig endures.

It's astonishing how many people love their pets as if they were family members, appreciating their personalities, extending their kindness and sustaining loving relationships with them, protecting them from harm, and going to great lengths to treat them when they are sick or injured, but then these people turn around and support and partake in the brutalization of other species by buying and eating animal products. If these people were to treat their housepets the way farm animals are treated, they would immediately be arrested and shunned by the public for their heartless cruelty.

"The greatness of a nation and its moral progress can be judged by the way its animals are treated."

≈✶ GANDHI

Many people are addicted to the "taste" of flesh foods, unaware that the taste they are really enjoying is the steak sauces and seasonings used in the preparation. These days there are many vegetarian "meat substitutes" available to those who crave this certain texture and taste, and if you use the same dressings and preparations, you will not be able to tell the difference. A shitake mushroom grilled and "sauced up" will satisfy most meat eaters. Veggie burgers taste much better than any flesh burger. It's hard to tell the difference between the two, and just think, there's no blood in my burger! Seitan and Tempeh are two meat substitutes that taste and feel very similar to meat and are becoming very popular.

If the great physiological and psychological damage we perpetrate by eating flesh is not reason enough for us to consider ending this malefic practice, maybe the following will provide some added incentive.

Before you order Veal Scaloppini again, here is something you might want to know. To bring that white flesh to your plate, a very sadistic operation takes place on the farm. The calf is pulled from its mother after birth. Cows are driven mad by the abduction of their offspring and have been known to kick holes in cement walls. The calf is chained and shackled to a tiny stall where the animal is unable to move, turn around or lie down comfortably. Frightened and alone, desperate to suck on anything and to feel the connection with its mother, this calf is forced to live in its own filth and excrement, is forced to spend its entire existence in the dark, is force-fed an artificial drug-laced diet, and intentionally is made to be anemic before its slaughter. Veal is torture.

Most of the industrialized farms, which make up the majority of farms, have cattle living in football field long row houses where the animals never see the light of day or touch their hoofs on the earth. They are kept on a steel grate their entire existence, which causes painful deformities and injuries to their hoofs and legs. They are fed and injected with drugs, steroids, antibiotics, and constantly sprayed with toxic pesticides in the course

of, their agonizing lives. The commonly sprayed pesticide toxaphene, according to the U.S. Environmental
Protection Agency, is so toxic that a few parts per billion
will dissolve the bones of an animal. This deadly poison
is absorbed into the flesh of these animals.

There are NO doctors or pharmaceutical experts
that can predict, in terms of the danger or "side effects,"
what happens when you mix two drugs together let alone
the ten to twenty pharmaceuticals with which these
cows are often fed and injected. These cattle are being
pumped with drugs their entire lives. However, scientists
do know that something called T.H.M.s (trihalometh-
anes) are formed when mixing drugs. THMs are a known
carcinogen.

The 3,000 doctors that make up The Physicians
Committee for Responsible Medicine estimate the annual
health care costs resulting directly from meat consumption to be somewhere between $23.6 billion and $61.4
billion.

Penicillin is commonly fed to and injected into farm
animals. Many human beings can die from an allergic
reaction to this commonly used drug. How much more
penicillin does the cow need compared to a human being?
Obviously a considerable amount more, considering that
cows are eight to ten times our size. Because of the unnatural bizarre environment these cattle (also chickens and
pigs) are raised in, the frequency of the drugging is quite
high. So there are extremely high doses of a drug that
can kill human beings in much smaller doses, frequently
administered to millions of farm animals that we commonly eat. There are no warnings to the public, no labels

listing the plethora of drugs that come with each pound of ground beef, chicken leg, slice of bacon or hotdog, and there is hardly an objection from the public.

Steroids and growth hormones, sadly enough, are being used by most all of today's professional and many amateur athletes. These performance enhancers turn average athletes into supermen and have reduced every baseball, basketball and football game into nothing but a pharmaceutical contest. These strength and performance enhancers are directly related to heart disease, strokes, and heart attacks. Anabolic steroids are implanted in the ears of cattle in the form of time release pellets. These hormones seep into the bloodstream and increase the hormone levels by two to five times. According to an article in the *National Food Review* (July–September 1989), over ninety-five percent of feedlot-raised cattle in the U.S. are currently being administered growth-inducing hormones.

Could the conclusion be made that most of our citizens are ingesting steroids on a daily basis? How does this affect the way we treat one another? Could the violence in our society have anything to do with the ingesting of steroids? Trial attorneys have been known to use the defense "my client was on steroids at the time of the crime."

I doubt even the heartiest meat eater on the planet would not be affected by the following. The FDA and the USDA allow and approve the following to be used as feed for farm animals. Chicken feces, cow feces, and ground up cardboard, cement dust, ammonia, "plastic hay," body parts of other chickens and cows, and IRRADIATED SEWAGE SLUDGE. They actually take sewage sludge and expose it to nuclear fallout (cesium 167, cobalt 60) and use it as feed.

The result, many people eat this poisoned flesh and die immediately, or a few days after ingestion. Our medical experts have the nerve to blame these deaths and violent seizures and sickness that meat eaters increasingly experience on salmonella or E. Coli bacteria, never mentioning the concentration of toxins, deadly pharmaceuticals, pesticides, steroids and growth hormones, or irradiated sewage sludge found in these animal products. *Would people knowingly ingest and pay for such a sickening array of ingredients, or is deception and misrepresentation necessary for profit?*

These sentient beings are treated with no dignity or compassion and live an agonizing-unnatural existence filled with dis-ease and physical pain. It is no wonder that few if any of our citizens are ever exposed to the brutal and cruel existence these animals endure, I wonder how many people would change their diet if they spent five minutes on the kill floor of a slaughterhouse amongst the screaming animals, chopped off heads, and rivers of blood.

Life on the factory farm is no better for chickens. They are commonly kept in two foot by two-foot cages, six to a cage. They have their beaks sawed off (an agonizing event), are driven insane by this torturous existence, often resorting to pecking each other's eyes out and

> *"Non-violence leads to the highest ethics, which is the goal of all evolution. Until we stop harming all other living beings, we are all still savages."*
>
> — THOMAS EDISON

killing one another. They are unable to move, their nails grow around the cages, and they too are fed a steady diet of antibiotics and pharmaceuticals along with poisoned and toxic feeds.

Our leaders speak about the violence on TV and in movies as being a main cause of the violence in our society. This violence that is portrayed on the screen is pretend violence utilizing actors playing roles and saying lines from a script. It may seem very real yet, these actors all go home intact and unharmed; it is pretend violence. Does it have an impact? There is a possibility that it does, and, according to some "experts," pretend violence does affect the way we treat each other. But the unseen, unrealizable murder and mayhem that goes on every day in these slaughterhouses is REAL VIOLENCE that makes a Freddy Krueger movie look like Sesame Street.

Many Americans are shocked at the heinous treatment of dogs in Korea and other dog eating countries. These dogs exist in the most deplorable and inhumane conditions and are often intentionally terrified before they are slaughtered to "make the meat taste better." Our population thinks it reprehensible and outrageously cruel to treat man's best friend with such indignity and cruelty, and those "dog-eaters" are viewed as barbaric and wicked human beings by our civilized society. Apparently, our "civilized" culture has the inside information on what are the proper animals to torture and slaughter and has no hesitation supporting the millions of daily murders that go on in our own slaughter houses.

Can any human being really appreciate what ten million daily killings entail? Do we have the capacity to feel for and understand the amount of pain and agony that is inflicted on these animals daily? Just because they are animals we have not met, does it mean it is all right to abuse and slaughter them? Does this have an effect on how we view the suffering of other human beings? Can we calculate the effects of this daily sadistic inhumanity and the impact it has on our population? No, it is quite obvious that we would be overwhelmed by our attempts to really appreciate all these issues, all the beings, and all the agonies endured. It is not possible for us.

Remember this is REAL violence, not make-believe… REAL VIOLENCE that takes place millions of times EACH DAY. Real violence has real consequences. The vibratory thrust of these daily holocausts hangs heavily over our populace and has grave repercussions for us all. Would anyone doubt that the cessation of torturing and killing animals would have a tremendously uplifting effect on our culture?

Niccolo Machiavelli, the Renaissance diplomat and tactician, when commenting on uncivilized tribes and their rituals reported the following:

> "Their ceremonies lacked neither pomp nor magnificence, but they added the extremely bloody and fierce act of sacrifice in which hordes of animals were killed. This savage aspect of them tended to make the participants savage too."

Remember that every time you buy a product you are voting. What does it say about our society that we in an overwhelming majority vote for and support this daily animal abuse? Do you want to continue voting this way because it "tastes good?"

You might want to ask yourself, "Is it really the taste of the meat I enjoy, or is it the texture, salt, pepper, spices, herbs, and other flavorings that I enjoy?" "Is it the emotional ties and familiarity to which I've grown so accustomed?" "Would I be doing myself and the rest of the world, including my family, a big favor by finding other comfort foods?"

If you have any doubt whether you can be as strong and powerful as you like on a vegetarian diet and the examples of the Herculean strength of nature's animals (rhinoceros, ox, horse, elephant, and gorilla, etc.) are not enough, here is a list of great human athletes that have left off the eating of animals:

CARL LEWIS: Maybe the greatest athlete ever, won a total of nine Olympic gold medals and numerous world championships. Held world records in the 100-meter dash and 400-meter relay. The one time "fastest man in the world" would consistently beat a field of drug-enhanced challengers. He may be the last pure track star of our time.

EDWIN MOSES: World and Olympic champion went eight years without losing a race in the 400-meter hurdles. He is possibly the most dominate athlete of his time. Sports Illustrated Athlete of the Year 1984.

BILL WALTON: Basketball player. He may be the most dominant collegiate center ever, winning four NCAA championships at UCLA. Walton went on to win NBA championships with the Portland Trail Blazers and the Boston Celtics.

MURRAY ROSE: Three-time gold medallist in the 1956 Olympics. Four years later came back to become the first man to retain his 400-meter freestyle title; he broke his own world record in the 400 and 1500 meter freestyle. Rose has been a vegetarian since he was two.

DON LALONDE: Professional Prizefighter. Light Heavy Weight Champion of the World.

ANDREAS CABLING: A Swedish bodybuilder who won the Mr. International title in 1980 and competed for 10 years at the highest level of body building competition.

DAVE SCOTT: Won the Ironman Triathlon four times.

ROY HILLIGAN: A vegetarian bodybuilder who won the Mr. America title.

STAN PRICE: A powerlifter who held the world record for bench press in his weight class.

BILL PEARL: World famous bodybuilder and lifting guru.

David Carter: Defensive lineman for the Chicago Bears.

Lauren Lovette: Principal Dancer, New York City Ballet.

According to Grecian lore, Milo of Croton, a Pythagorean disciple, was a legendary wrestler who never lost a match. He was a victor in five successive Olympiads in the sixth century BC, and the story goes that he was never brought to his knees.

This list can go on a lot longer, but the point is well made. Whether it is the pure strength, physical toughness, endurance, skill, speed, or a combination of them all, this list of great athlete's is evidence enough that vegetarians lose nothing by leaving off the eating of animals.

I am convinced that as soon as one major athlete recognizes the benefits of not just vegetarianism or veganism, but raw foodism and begins to abide by the Laws of Nature, other athletes will quickly follow.

Fish

There are many people who call themselves vegetarians and continue to eat fish. I have yet to see a plant grow a fish. I have often heard people who come across an unpleasant odor exclaim with disgust and offensive distaste, "It smells like fish in here." I do not know too many people who find the look or smell of fish, let alone the scaly texture, appealing or inviting, not to mention appetizing. Walking by a fishery on the pier can be a sickening experience if you do not have some heavy cloth to press against your nose to protect you from the gag-inducing, putrid stench. If someone were to plunk a dead fish into your lap right now, what would your initial, instinctive reaction be?

In spite of our natural aversion to the presence of dead fish, we are happy to order our well cooked and carefully prepared "filet of sole." It really is quite an amazing trick we play on ourselves, and it makes me wonder

if there is no limit to what we might eat if it were presented in the right way. This stinking fish we want to get
away from as fast as possible somehow becomes an item
we want on our dinner plate, and we gladly pay for it.
Conversely, if someone threw an apple on your lap . . . you
might thank them.

The Center for Disease Control claims an average of
325,000 reports of food poisoning from fish each year. If that
is what is reported, one has to wonder how many more poisonings go unreported. Due to our heavily polluted oceans,
lakes, and rivers, most fish contain mercury, an extremely
toxic metal substance that can destroy the nervous system
and cause grave illness. There are only a few areas where fish
are not living in mercury-tainted waters.

In addition to mercury, it is more than common that
the fish on our plates have large amounts of PCB's. A
synthetic liquid used for industrial purposes, this baneful
carcinogen was outlawed in 1976. A six-month investigation done by Consumers Union revealed that "by far the
biggest source of PCB's in the human diet is fish" and "the
PCB's you eat today will be with you for decades into the
future." Ingesting PCB's causes reduced sperm counts in
men and may be directly related to birth defects.

Many environmental experts and oceanographers
have given a stern warning to humanity about the over-
fishing that is destroying the homeostasis of our oceans.
High tech industrial fishing methods, including sonar
and spotting planes, have enabled commercial fishers to
vacuum up eighty to ninety percent of entire fish popula-
tions in one year's time. The United Nations has reported
that all seventeen major fishing areas on our planet have

either reached or exceeded their natural limits. Just as we are clear cutting and annihilating our rainforests, we are razing and pillaging our oceans. Two of our most precious resources are being devastated because we insist on an animal-based diet. A shocking fact (from The Pew Environment group 2008) and another reason to stop eating animals is that one-third of all caught fish are turned into fish-meal for livestock.

If our oceans make up seventy percent of our planet and they are being destroyed and polluted, how does that impact on the rest of our environment?

Land usage and starving children

Besides wreaking havoc on our bodies and compromising our conscience, our animal-based diet is a significant factor in the destruction of our planet and also one of the main contributing factors in the hunger and starvation of millions.

From a Sierra Club article (1999):

"A December 1997 report prepared for Iowa Senator Tom Harkin (D), who sits on the Senate Committee on Agriculture, says that animal waste is the largest contributor to pollution in 60 percent of the rivers and streams classified as 'impaired' by the Environmental Protection Agency. According to the same report, the United States generates 1.4 billion tons of animal manure every year-130 times more than the annual production of human waste. Cattle manure leads the list at 1.2 billion tons, followed by pig manure at 116 million tons, and chicken manure at 14 million tons."

> *"I tremble for my species when I reflect that God is just."*
>
> ⇒✶ THOMAS JEFFERSON

One-third of the world's total grain production goes to feed cattle. Less than half of the farm acreage in this country is now used to grow food for people. The livestock population of the U.S. consumes enough grains and soybeans to feed the American population five times over. The livestock population gets over eighty percent of the corn and ninety-five percent of the oats we grow. One half of our water supply goes to cattle farming. Cattle outweigh human beings on the planet two to one. Yet we do not hear politicians or UN representatives address this growing population disaster, this locust-like swarm of cattle that is ravaging our planet; yet they continue to warn us of human overpopulation on a daily basis.

The over one billion cattle on this planet produce over one-fifth of the environmentally devastating methane gas, which may be destroying our ozone layer.

At the turn of the nineteenth century, American farmland had a topsoil that averaged twenty-one inches in depth. Today only six inches remain. The meat industry is responsible for over eighty-five percent of the topsoil erosion in this country.

In 1984, when thousands of people in Ethiopia were dying daily from starvation, that country continued to export grain and feed to European countries as cattle feed. There are currently millions of acres of third world countries being exclusively used to produce feed for European cattle while many of their people starve to death.

Malnutrition is the principle cause of death in many third world countries. In many of these countries' twenty-five percent of the population dies before the age of four. Guatemala exports forty million pounds of beef to the United States while seventy-five percent of their children under the age of five are undernourished. The conditions in Costa Rica and the rest of Central America are not much better.

This hunger and suffering that runs rampant throughout our world are not caused by any defect of nature. The pain, starvation, and death are caused by human beings who must be uninformed, disinterested, arrogant, greedy, or all of the above.

"More than twenty-five percent of the forests in Central America have been cleared for pasture land, and most cattle produced is exported to developing countries for use in fast food hamburgers."

≋✿ COSTA RICA
RAINFOREST OUTWARD
BOUND SCHOOL, 1996

Every three seconds, a child dies of starvation.

Yet we continue to prioritize the feeding of livestock. It is quite clear that by living the way we presently do, that by making the food choices we presently make in our "civilized" countries, we are directly contributing to the savagery and brutality of mass starvation.

The most precious lands on our planet are being systematically destroyed so we can have cheap hamburgers. Tropical rainforests across the globe are being annihilated to graze cattle, setting off a long and dangerous domino effect of ecological and environmental destruction.

The current rate of species extinction is 1000 per year, and most of that is directly related to the destruction of these incredibly lush and vibrant rainforests that are an essential part of our planet's well being.

Mexico and Central America used to be covered by 160,000 square miles of tropical rainforests; they now are down to under 40,000 square miles as the clear-cutting for cattle pastures continues. These forests have taken thousands of years to develop and are a major part of our eco-system. If this destruction continues, we may never recover.

Francis Moore Lappe, the author of the environmental classic *Diet for a Small Planet*, described how Caterpillar tractors are razing and annihilating the Latin American rainforests. "Gargantuan 35 ton D-9s mounted with angle plows weighing 2,500 pounds each bulldoze the forest at 2,700 yards an hour uprooting everything in sight." For every quarter pound hamburger that comes from a steer raised in Central and South America, it is necessary to destroy approximately 165 pounds of living matter.

In Plato's *Republic*, Socrates claims that people should avoid things "not required by any natural want." Certainly, it is clear that eating animals is a habit we have taken on, but NOT a natural want. Socrates goes on to have the following dialogue with Glaucon.

SOCRATES: And there will be animals of many
   other kinds, if people eat them?

GLAUCON: Certainly.

SOCRATES: And living this way we shall have
   a much greater need of physicians than
   before?

GLAUCON: Much greater.

SOCRATES: And the country which was enough
   to support

the original inhabitants will be too small now
   and not enough?

GLAUCON: Quite true

SOCRATES: Then a slice of our neighbors land
   will be wanted by us for pasture and tillage,
   and they will want a slice of ours, if, like
   ourselves, they exceed the limit of necessity
   and give themselves up to the unlimited
   accumulation of wealth?

GLAUCON: That, Socrates, will be inevitable.

SOCRATES: And so we shall go to war, Glaucon.
   Shall we not?

GLAUCON: Most certainly.

—Plato, *The Republic* II, 373 BC

"You cannot do wrong without suffering wrong."

≡≍ EMERSON

   This war that Plato and Socrates had foreseen has been intensely raging in and around us, making victims of all who live in such a numbed-out, violent world. The very food we destroy our planet to create is the very food that is ravaging our bodies and destroying our physical health and numbing our abilities to feel. Sleeping humanity has become a growing cancer. Is it any wonder the very societies that are most deadly to the environment experience cancer and disease at such an alarming rate? As above, so below. We have no regard for nature and, in turn, less regard for ourselves. How can health and harmony exist when we live in such utter **IGNORANCE** and promote the daily violence against our animals, environment, and starving masses of humanity by purchasing these products of cruelty?

"The vegetarian movement ought to fill the souls of those who have, at heart the realization of God's Kingdom upon earth."

≈✴ LEO TOLSTOY

For some reason "civilized" humanity believes itself to be above the laws that govern our world. Such arrogance is not held by any indigenous peoples or "uncivilized" tribes. Native Americans could not understand the idea of "owning land" as they felt that they were part of the Earth and that in fact, the Earth owned them. Hunting did exist among these people, but they had great reverence for the animal that gave its life so they could live. They never took more than they needed and always viewed themselves as A PART of creation, NOT the epitome or "Lord of Nature" that modern man deems himself. When laws are broken, there are penalties to pay.

These "uncivilized" people, like animals in nature, do not kill out of hatred or try to control, dominate, enslave, or torture other species. They kill for survival and take what is needed, thus, the balance in the natural world is never threatened by their actions. The neurotic behavior of trying to control nature has bred a world with a civilization filled with frightened, desperate, depressed, and insatiable people on the brink of oblivion. You can make a conscious choice to no longer support this cycle of insanity. Remember you are either part of the solution or part of the problem.

Many great teachers have reminded us of our interconnectedness with other beings, yet, few of us ever consider this teaching when sitting down to eat. And we will continue to suffer as we continue to create suffering. Of course, the opposite is a possibility if you choose.

I hope you take some time to give some deep consideration to these issues and join the long list of compassionate and brilliant individuals throughout history who have understood the necessity of non-violence. I can promise you that the quality of your health will be enhanced dramatically by leaving off the eating of animals, and you will be doing a great service to our planet by doing so and, in turn, a great service to yourself.

> There was a time, the golden age we call it,
> happy in fruits and herbs, when no men tainted
> their lips with blood, and birds went flying safely
> through the air, and in the fields rabbits
> wandered
> unfrightened, and no fish was ever
> hooked by its own credulity: All things
> were free from treachery and fear and canning,
> and all was peaceful. But some innovator,

a good-for-nothing whoever he was, decided,
in envy, that what lions ate was better,
stuffed meat into his belly like a furnace,
and paved the way for crime . . .
One crime leads to another.

—Pythagoras from Ovid's *Metamorphosis*

Gandhi's influence on our global society cannot yet be entirely counted as the ripples of his knowledge, courage and veracity continue to impact and influence those leaders and followers who strive for decency. Ghandi's words and actions continue to impact men who search for truth and stand as an eternal example of man's appropriate stature. I find the following excerpt from this great, perceptive and loving being a wonderful way to sum up this chapter.

Speech delivered by Gandhi at a Social Meeting organized by the London Vegetarian Society, November 20, 1931:

> "I used to attend debates that were held between vegetarians. Then vegetarians had a habit of talking of nothing but food and disease. I feel that is the worst way of going about the business. It is those persons who become vegetarians because they are suffering from some disease or other who largely fall back. I discovered that for remaining staunch to vegetarianism a man requires a moral basis.
>
> For me, that was a great discovery in my search after truth. At an early age, I found that

a selfish basis would not serve the purpose of taking a man higher and higher along the paths of evolution. What was required was an altruistic purpose. I found also that several vegetarians found it impossible to remain vegetarians because they had made food a fetish and because they thought that by becoming vegetarians they could eat as much as they liked. Of course, those people could not possibly keep their health.

Observing along these lines, I saw that a man should eat sparingly and now and then fast. I discovered that in order to keep healthy, it was necessary to cut down the quantity of your food and reduce the number of meals. Become moderate, err on the side of less, rather than on the side of more.

What I want to bring to your notice is that vegetarians need to be tolerant if they want to convert others to vegetarianism. Adopt a little humility. We should appeal to the moral sense of the people who do not see eye to eye with us. If a vegetarian became ill, and a doctor prescribed beef tea, then I would not call him a vegetarian. A vegetarian is made of sterner stuff. Why? Because it is for the building of the spirit and not of the body. Therefore vegetarians should have that moral basis—that a man was not born a carnivorous animal, but born to live on the fruits and herbs that the earth grows. If anybody said that I should die if I did not take beef-tea or mutton, even on medical advice, I would prefer death. That is the basis of my vegetarianism.

There must be a definite reason for our making that change in our lives, from our adopting habits and customs different from society, even though sometimes that change may offend those nearest and dearest to us. Not for the world should you sacrifice a moral principle. The only basis for having a vegetarian society and proclaiming a vegetarian principle is and must be, a moral one.

Therefore, I thought that during the few minutes which I give myself the privilege of addressing you, I would just emphasize the moral basis of vegetarianism. And I would say that I have found from my own experience and the experience of thousands of friends and companions, that they find satisfaction from the moral basis they have chosen for sustaining vegetarianism."

—Excerpt from *The Moral Basis of Vegetarianism* by Mohandas Karamchand (Mahatma) Gandhi

DAIRY PRODUCTS

How many times have we heard the phrase "Milk is a Natural?" That is quite a broad statement. First of all what kind of milk is being considered, and second of all natural for whom? Certainly dog milk is natural for puppies, cat milk is natural for kittens, and cow milk is natural for calves. It's difficult to argue this fact, as the nursing of these mammals is as natural and instinctive as any act in nature. No sane individual would argue this fact. However, when being told that the milk of a one thousand pound animal is a "natural" for human consumption, the true thinker might raise an eyebrow or two.

Imagine if you saw people in a cow pasture drop to their knees and start sucking on a cow's teat. What would your response be? Surprise? ... shock? ... disbelief? You might even be disgusted, but pour yourself a glass of the same stuff from a cardboard container and all of a sudden the shock and disgust disappear.

We are the only species on the planet that drinks the milk of another species.

Drinking the milk of this bovine beast is a bizarre and highly unnatural act. What could be more unnatural than this peculiar habit of attempting to nourish ourselves with another species' milk? When you go against the Laws of Nature, you will pay the price.

This corrupt act is made worse by the cooking or "pasteurization" process that all of our dairy products go through. The high temperatures destroy and coagulate most all of the nutrients we might be able to utilize and make this already troublesome food that much more difficult to digest.

Of all the unconscious acts we perform against our health and well being, the ingestion of dairy products is right up near the top in terms of dis-ease producing habits.

Cow's milk has a very specific natural function to feed the offspring of these large animals. Calves are usually born at around 50 to 60 pounds. In a month and a half they double in size, and in one year's time they grow to an amazing 1000 pounds or more, nurtured solely on the milk of the mother. This incredible growth spurt is created by the nutrients and hormones in this milk.

It is plain to see that milk is the essential food of mammals' offspring. It IS a "natural" in this respect. It is necessary and wholesome and provides newborns with the proper nutrition to build and maintain their bodies without the help of any other food. It is nature's perfect food for the offspring of the designated species. It is important to note that . . . .

No full-grown mammal in nature consumes any milk.

There are no full grown cows drinking cows' milk. This is another inarguable fact. You cannot find a mature animal in nature trying to suckle its mother. You certainly would spend the rest of your life trying to find a full-grown mammal approaching the mother of another species to drink her milk.

Drinking the milk of a cow is a bizarre act.

One of our distinct human attributes is the ability to reason. Why would any full grown, reasonable human being partake in the ingesting of milk designed for the offspring of a completely different species and think it advantageous to their health? The answer is your pick: Advertising or brainwashing.

The dairy council is one of the more powerful lobbies in Washington and has tremendous influence in setting public policy on Capitol Hill. In 1998, the dairy industry spent 90 million dollars on their ubiquitous mustache campaign, paying celebrities and athletes to promote this dis-ease producer. Not only did they get our president to do one of their advertisements, but, shockingly, the highest-ranking health official in the land, Donna Shalala, the Secretary of Health and Human Services, appeared with the "milk-stache" in Health Magazine. That's no different from our Attorney General advertising for the Mafia.

Human babies have the enzymes rennin and lactase in their bodies up until the age of three to four years old. These two enzymes are necessary for the digestion of human breast milk. Once the child begins to form teeth, the rennin and lactase are no longer produced, and he or she is weaned and begins to eat solid food, no longer relying on milk. This is nature's plan. Our Dairy Council and "health experts" have different plans.

If the natural hormonal balance in cow's milk, this food we so commonly and thoughtlessly consume, is great enough to support such intense growth spurts for the calf in one years time, is it possible that this food could be harmful and dis-ease producing in a human body? When a male human being is born at seven to ten pounds and a female human being at only a few pounds lighter, it takes at least eighteen years for them to reach full maturity. This is obviously a totally different growth rate than that of a cow. What problems are created when human beings are fed these daily doses of animal food with all its powerful, bovine designed hormones?

Putting cow's milk in a human body is no different than putting rocket fuel in your family car, Your car is going to have some serious problems running on a fuel designed for a totally different type of machine. The results of both inappropriate fuel choices are disastrous. Our society suffers greatly from this outlandish and accepted practice of feeding on the milk of another species.

Dairy products are one of the most dis-ease producing foods on the planet.

There is an enzyme in cow's milk called casein. Casein is used to make one of the strongest wood bonding glues on the planet. This gooey sticky substance wreaks havoc in the human digestive tract. It adheres to the walls of the intestinal tract unable to be broken down and hardens, creating a wall of intestinal plaque which significantly impairs the body's ability to absorb the needed nutrients from other foods we eat. Of course, if your body does not absorb what is needed, your appetite will continue to grow, no matter how much food you ingest. The opposite is also true. If the intestinal tract is clean and the body able to absorb the needed nutrients, very small meals will be incredibly satiating. Ingesting dairy products is one of the most counterproductive things one can do when trying to lose weight.

Because of the large doses of dairy products ingested by our children, their hormonal balance is gravely affected, which often leads to what doctors call "behavioral diseases."

There are over three million children in the U.S. taking Ritalin and other brain-numbing, dis-ease-producing drugs, which is a horrifying fact. Many adolescent girls reach puberty prematurely, and a majority of children and teenagers suffer and battle with weight problems and acne due to milk poisoning. Dr. Norman Walker, an advocate of natural living who lived 109 years, did extensive studies on the effects of cow's milk on human glands and found that the thyroid gland can be greatly damaged by the casein found in dairy products.

Millions of children are being dangerously drugged for a condition known as asthma, a condition directly related to dairy products and their clogging, restrictive effects on the lungs and air passages. What a disastrous event to entrap our children in a lifelong dependence on daily drugging, steroids, inhalers, and then give them the crippling news that they have "incurable" dis-ease. Of course adults are also directly affected by this unnatural feeding; however, a grown man or woman has the opportunity to question and decide for him or herself. Our children are completely dependent on us, and if we have not taken the time to question what we have been told, our children are doomed to a life of dis-ease and pharmaceutical dependency.

Is it possible that the vast influx of foreign hormones we commonly ingest is affecting our glandular system and our hormonal homeostasis? Is it possible that the deep depressions, the emotional instabilities, and the mood swings our society increasingly suffers from are related to or even caused by these cow hormones?

We have all heard of those who are allergic to cow's milk and those who are "lactose intolerant." The fact is, we are ALL allergic to cow's milk. Some of us just have a more acute response to this human toxin. Of course, salesmen have provided us with treatments and products that can help us "overcome and tolerate" our natural intolerance.

Once again industry, ignorant and often greedy "health experts," and hapless celebrities are responsible for promoting the madness that dairy products are "good for you." But we are responsible for believing them.

Besides creating an extremely acid condition in our bodies, clogging arteries, disrupting and impeding digestion, weakening bones, wreaking havoc on our hormonal systems, causing painful headaches, earaches, and infections, and contributing to many allergies, cow's milk is a major contributing factor to obesity.

There are over 65 million people suffering from obesity in this country and hardly a word from the AMA, HMOs, hospitals, or doctors about the heinous effects of this "food."

Calcium

We have been told over and over again that dairy products are important to build strong bones and that we need the calcium that dairy products provide. Young and old alike are told this baseless lie, and the belief is so entrenched in our day to day "thinking" that it is a great challenge to find a dairy-free household in this country. If dairy products build strong bones and prevent osteoporosis, why is it that the number one consumer of dairy products, the United States, has the highest rate of osteoporosis? If dairy products prevent osteoporosis and we consume such massive amounts, should we not have the strongest, healthiest bones?

Nathan Pritikin did a study on the Bantu tribe of Africa. Hundreds of women who birthed an average of nine babies each and breast fed them all were found to have NO cases of osteoporosis, and they ingested NO dairy products. They never lost a tooth and rarely broke a bone. The National Dairy Council recommends that we ingest 1200 milligrams a day of calcium. The Bantu's average intake of calcium is 350 milligrams.

Eskimos take in more than 2,000 milligrams a day of calcium and suffer from one of the highest rates of osteoporosis in the world. This sad condition has coincided directly with the infection of "civilization" with all its processed, refined foods.

Calcium works as a neutralizing agent in the body, offsetting acid conditions that occur from improper feeding. Many people are suffering from calcium deficiencies because their bodies are in a constant acid state, thus the body's calcium supply is leeched from the bones to neutralize the acidity in the bloodstream and repeatedly exhausted. LESS consumption of animal products would increase the availability of calcium in the body. Once again, a glance over at the natural world shows us that there are no animals in nature with calcium deficiencies. Gorillas, rhinos, horses, oxen, all incredibly powerful animals with huge Herculean bodies, eat nothing but plant life and have the strongest bones on the planet.

Years ago, I was involved in a motorcycle accident. I was hit by a car from behind and had my four hundred and fifty pound, motorcycle drop, with the added force of momentum, down on my leg and pin me to the cobblestone street. I was bleeding and in great pain but, despite the force of the direct impact on my leg, there was no break. The ambulance attendants were amazed I was able to walk and were convinced the leg must be broken. It was not. I went back to work after the accident.

If you are concerned about getting enough calcium, you'll have nothing to worry about if you are eating mostly raw foods. Fruits, green leafy vegetables, seeds, and nuts contain calcium that is easily assimilated. Sesame seeds have the highest concentration of calcium in any food. Seaweed such as dulse and kelp are also great sources of calcium. All of these foods promote an alkaline, non-acidic state in the body.

In 1983, the Journal of Clinical Nutrition did a massive study on the health and bone densities of vegetarians versus meat-eaters. Here are their results:

By the age of 65:

- Meat eating men had an average 4% more measurable bone loss than vegetarians.
- Meat eating women had an average 17% more bone loss than vegetarian women.
- Meat eating women had lost 35% bone mass.

There have yet to be any studies done on the bones of raw foodists, but we can take a look at the animal raw foodists in nature and do our own study. We can see quite clearly that osteoporosis simply does not exist for those that live in accordance with nature and their natural instincts.

If the information above is not impetus enough for you to stop or at least question ingesting dairy products, maybe the following will provide more compelling evidence.

There are many women in this country who are intimidated into taking artificial hormones upon reaching menopause. Again, the medical message is, "Nature has made a mistake, and we can help you." This time of life has become such a difficulty for women because the body is in such turmoil. Hormonal imbalances are the rule in our society due to our maligned or nonexistent health practices. Uncivilized tribal women and other mammals go through this same change and experience little to no debilitating upset in their system or loss of bone density.

Many of these hormonal treatments significantly increase the risk of cancer and cause many more problems than the symptoms they mask. If you are concerned about your bone density, weight training is an extremely effective way to maintain or increase your bone density no matter what age you may be. There is no need to bother with any of the hundreds of toxic supplements and calcium drinks (many filled with whey and other industrial wastes) on the market. Eat according to the Laws of Nature and exercise.

BGH (Bovine growth hormone)

We have reviewed the massive drugging that farm animals endure as they are fed and injected with antibiotics, steroids, tetracycline, penicillin and sprayed with insecticides. We have gone over the disgustingly shocking array of feeds that they are forced to ingest, including irradiated sewer sludge. It is no secret that most of these poisons are present in the milk of these abused animals.

Agent Orange (the deadly nerve gas used in the Vietnam War) and glyphosate (the main ingredient in

Roundup, which, according to *Scientific American* "can kill human cells"), is now responsible for the introduction of the frightening and perhaps apocalyptic technology know as genetically modified foods, has introduced a new product to the American consumer.

Considering that we spend close to fifty million tax-payer dollars a year in this country storing excess dairy products that will never be used and literally paying farmers subsidies NOT to produce milk, the need for a substance to make a cow produce more milk is certainly not a priority and plainly unreasonable. Making money, however, can affect reason.

Monsanto has convinced many farmers and corporations of the benefits of having each of their cows produce three to four times as much milk. Money has changed hands, deals have been struck, the FDA, our so-called watchdog agency, approved the use of BGH in 1990, and the madness continues.

According to USDA Agricultural Statistics, in 1960 an average cow produced 3.5 tons of milk per year; in 1990 as hormones and steroids were increasingly introduced, a single cow produced 7.4 tons of milk per year. After FDA approval of Bovine Growth Hormone, the average cow, in 1995, went on to produce 8.2 tons per year. According to the Associated Press (9/20/96), some BGH treated cows have gone on to produce 30 tons of milk in one year, more than 10 times their natural capacity.

Bovine Growth Hormone wreaks havoc on these animals causing their udders to painfully double in size resulting in painful infections and inflammation. According to experts, BGH works like the street drug crack (concentrated cocaine) on a cow. It causes increased heart rate, hypersensitivity, and a tremendous strain on the nervous system. A mature cow weighs anywhere from 1000 to 1200 pounds. If this hormone works like "crack" on a 1200 pound animal, how does it work on your seven-pound baby? Or a 200-pound man? Or your eight-year-old daughter or son?

In the last ten years, we have been increasingly told of a mysterious and new disease called SIDS: Sudden Infant Death Syndrome. Doctors and pediatric experts have continually professed these babies are dying by asphyxiation, choking and suffocating on their blankets and pillows, as if blankets and pillows are a new introduction to an infant's life. Because of these stern warnings to parents to "make your children sleep on their backs," there are a plethora of products and devices on the market to force your child to sleep in unnatural ways. There is no mystery to the rise in infant mortality to those who know of the malefic pharmaceutical cocktail laced with antibiotics, pesticides, and Bovine Growth Hormone we constantly and unknowingly put in our baby's bottle. Add to this the increasingly poisonous and lethal DPT vaccinations regularly administered to newborns that we accept and oversee as traditional medical "solutions."

Dairy substitutes

If you are concerned and panicking over the loss of your beloved milk and ice cream, I have some good news for you. There are some wonderful, easy to make substitutes for both of these products.

Almond milk is a wonderfully delicious substitute for cow's milk and takes about thirty seconds to prepare. You need some blanched almonds, a handful or so, and some water in a blender. The more you blend this, the more it looks like milk If you want, simply use a strainer to remove any nut pulp. It looks like milk but tastes a lot better and is easily digestible and quite nutritious.

For ice cream, you can peel some bananas and put them in the freezer. Once frozen, place them in a food processor, and you will have the richest, sweetest ice cream imaginable. Of course, you can add strawberries or blueberries or any other kind of fruit you wish. Try a little raw almond butter or tahini mixed in; it's delicious.

If you love butter, there is not much difference in consistency (plus the benefit of added flavor) when using an avocado instead. In fact avocado toast is now a popular "thing."

If you are a cheese addict, it is a good bet you are a salt addict as well, as cheese without the added salt is tasteless. There is an inordinate amount of salt contained in all cheeses. Cheese is a densely concentrated dairy product loaded with cholesterol, saturated fat, and the poisonous sodium chloride (salt).

Cheese used to be my favorite food. I included it in most of my meals and actually used to eat bars of mozzarella as snacks. After a year of going without this food, I allowed myself to taste just a bit and really expected to enjoy it. I literally had to spit it out and rinse my mouth

repeatedly to prevent myself from gagging. It felt like
I had a mouthful of salt and fat. I do not miss it, and
neither will you once you reestablish your natural body
and allow your taste buds to re-sensitize. Take a look at
some raw food preparation books or You Tube "raw vegan
cheese" online to see more alternatives. Raw cashew
cheese is delicious. There is also a product on the market
made from cooked arrowroot that looks a lot and tastes a
lot like cheese. The brand name is Daiya.

Eggs

What is an egg? . . . A putrefied chicken embryo. Of all
animal products, eggs have the highest percentage of cholesterol, a fact that the egg producers have taken criminal
efforts to hide. In the early seventies, the American Heart
Association reported on the baneful effects of cholesterol and cited eggs as a food to avoid. The National
Commission on Egg Nutrition was formed by these egg
selling companies specifically to challenge these claims.
Their organization's name gives the illusion of an impar-
tial government agency which supposedly gives the facts
on eggs. Hardly! The NCEN spent large sums of money
advertising in major newspapers stating: "There is absolutely no scientific evidence that eating eggs, even in
quantity, will increase the risk of heart attack."

The American Heart Association, armed with all the
necessary evidence, claimed that this was "false, deceptive, misleading advertising" and asked the Federal Trade
Commission to intervene. After considering the evidence,

the FTC filed a formal complaint against the National Commission on Egg Nutrition and its advertising agency. A lengthy court battle ensued, and the NCEN claimed they were exercising their right of "free speech" by advertising the benefits of eggs. The judge did not buy it and ruled that the statements made were "false, misleading, deceptive, and unfair."

Thirty years later these hucksters are still at it, spending millions of dollars "educating the public" and doing studies that "prove" eggs are good for you and "necessary" for your well being. One of their research tricks is to find people that have extremely high levels of cholesterol to use in their studies. When the body is saturated with cholesterol, additional cholesterol is not going to create a significant increase. Measuring the increase in cholesterol after eating an egg in these individuals produces an insignificant or negligible difference. By seeking out cholesterol-saturated subjects they can guarantee their studies will get the desired result that eggs do not "significantly increase blood cholesterol."

The egg producers continue to claim that we need cholesterol in our bodies. This is actually true, but once again the difference between the cholesterol our cells produce and the cholesterol found in eggs and animal products is of a COMPLETELY different nature. There is absolutely NO need for a human body to seek outside sources of cholesterol. The Task Force to the American Society of Clinical Nutrition states that "there is no known evidence that low cholesterol diets are harmful, or that dietary cholesterol is an essential nutrient in any human condition."

Eggs are extremely acidic and contain large amounts of sulfur. Sulfur has a pungent odor and has a seriously disruptive effect on the digestive system.

The abuse continues on the chicken farms with five to six chickens living in two-foot square pens and in stacks living on top of one another so they're forced to live in constant filth and excrement contaminated quarters. Because they are unable to move around, their bones become weak and brittle. They are driven insane by their cramped quarters and the denial of their natural instincts to bathe and build nests.

They too are exposed to an excess of hormones, antibiotics, and pesticides. Residues of these substances are extant and prevalent in the eggs of these tortured beings.

These last two chapters contain all the vital reasons to give up our animal-based diet. Remember, health does not have so much to do with what you put into your body compared to what you do not put into your body. Try a week or two on a vegan (no animal products) diet and see for yourself if you do not feel better. The next chapter contains all the knowledge you will ever need to know concerning how to feed yourself.

EATING ACCORDING TO THE LAWS OF NATURE

It is plain to see that the mass confusion that exists concerning what is the healthiest way to eat continues to grow. Expert after expert comes out with book after book promoting a plethora of treatments and revealing "new" methods and diet plans, including stapling stomachs, "exercise in a bottle," and deadly diet pills. Yet there is now 160 million obese or overweight people in this country, America has the largest population of overweight people in the world. 350,000 people have heart by-pass operations every year. According to the CDC more than 795,000 American citizens have a stroke each year and the numbers are climbing much like the number of new drugs that are dispensed year after year. The demand for the new stuff is created by the glaringly obvious, yet often not recognized, fact that NONE of the old stuff works. When the blind lead the blind both end up in a ditch.

Of course, coming up with an unaffected and unbiased opinion or perspective on the subject of nutrition is close to impossible with the inundation of information and "facts" we are exposed to regarding this subject. Because our eating habits are so emotionally and sensory based ("but it tastes so good") we are biased, hypersensitive, and threatened by the thought of having our comfort foods taken away from us. The cultural influence that one experiences in this or any civilized country are powerful and ubiquitous. The misinformation concerning human feeding habits is spread by advertising, false beliefs, and cultural folklore. The result is a society steeped in disease and confusion. If we want something new and better, we must be willing to give up the old.

Most people prefer their habits to the truth, even if those habits are killing them.

It is difficult to imagine an entirely new way of living. It takes real effort and an adventurous spirit to journey into the unknown and to relinquish the beliefs and habits that have kept us so comfortable, and so sick. It is scary and unfamiliar to clean off our mental shelves and make room for some new possibilities, but it is also the ONLY way we can grow.

A clear mind and a willingness to be objective are necessary requirements to find some authentic, reliable, and unbiased answers to the existing confusion concerning proper nutrition.

Nature never says one thing and wisdom another.

Nature is a wonderful teacher and always present with her lessons. There is a perpetual cyclical rhythm to our universe that is so beautifully and mysteriously maintained. There is an invisible though constant force at work to keep our atmosphere in precise balance in terms of the mixture of Oxygen, Nitrogen, Carbon dioxide, etc., that keeps us all alive. To regulate the temperature and to keep the sunshine in abundance where it is needed. Animals in nature have built-in instincts and tendencies that keep them alive and flourishing wherever man does not interfere or destroy nature's balance. We too have these built-in programs that were designed to guide us. The problem is that our instincts are buried under a myriad of untruths and misinformation to which we have grown so accustomed that our contact with our instincts has been severely compromised, if not fully erased.

Whether one believes in God or not, it is quite difficult to deny that a magnificent intelligence IS at work all around us as well as inside of us. There is an obvious balance to our universe. Why is it then that we human beings suffer so much dis-ease? Could it be that we live unbalanced, inharmonious lives that interrupt and distort nature's intent?

There is a universal organization. Fred Hoyle, the British astronomer and founder of the Institute for Theoretical Astronomy at Cambridge University, says that the probability of wisps of gas and specks of clay becoming alive is madly improbable and "about as likely

as assembling a Boeing 747 by sending a whirling tor-
nado into a junkyard." Humanity seems so puffed up
with our technological advancements and achieve-
ments that we lack the necessary humility to recognize
and respect nature's design. The lack of recognition and
flagrant disrespect for this organizational force and its
incomprehensible wisdom is at the core of our difficulties
and confusion.

Nature and the creative energy behind it is ultimately
the greatest force known to man. There is NOTHING
that man can build or produce that nature cannot do
away with swiftly and completely. Those that taunt and
disrespect nature find this out immediately and often pay
with their lives.

Man has a tremendous ego that insists it can overcome
nature. Whether it is building an "unsinkable ship" (Titanic)
or "earthquake-proof" buildings, devising a pill that will
"allow you to go without sleep," creating drugs that will
"burn fat" while you lie on your couch, or manufacturing
"convenience foods" (what's more convenient than a banana,
or an apple?) man's list of attempts to go against nature are
long and laughable and the results disastrous. At the same
time, by studying and working WITH nature's dynamics,
we have been able to build flying machines, automobiles, and
many extraordinary inventions.

The Wright brothers and the earliest designers of
aviators (including Leonardo Da Vinci) studied diligently
the flight of birds and the relationship between the air
and wings, including speed, weight, and the properties of
lift that already existed in nature. Through this respectful
study of nature, they were able to imitate, closely enough,

the necessary properties needed for flight. Working WITH Nature's Laws was the only way flight was realized. Such inventions, created by the study of nature and natural laws, have provided us with a once unimaginable lifestyle.

Although airplane technology is continually advancing, it is still not as effective as the hummingbirds or eagle's astounding capabilities. Birds rarely crash or fall out of the sky uncontrollably, yet hundreds of people die each year in aviation crashes. There is no jet airplane in the world that can dive like a hawk or corner like a sparrow, and there may never be.

No matter how sophisticated the plane, every sane pilot in the world recognizes and fully respects nature's force and works with the Laws of Nature NOT against them.

Throughout the ages, there have been and will continue to be those human beings that contend that they know better and are wiser than nature. They insist on working against nature, attempting to dominate and/or control it, and refusing to recognize the inherent wisdom and force of the natural world. Many of these arrogant human beings hold positions of respect and are regarded with great esteem. These are the shortsighted "health experts" and "scientists" that insist that nature has made mistakes, and they do a great job convincing uninformed minds that they have improved on nature's ways.

In laboratories stocked with the latest technological advances and measuring devices, scientists insist on taking their lab results and computer readouts as the paramount law, ignoring the most simple and obvious facts that are evident in the natural world. Our *society creates havoc by manufacturing and promoting a toxic diet and then insisting that the answers to the diseases created must be found in a laboratory.* This creates the illusion we have today that health is a complicated issue that only can be understood by the select and highly "educated" scientists.

High-tech analysis of the human body and the nutrients and components of our food often leads to false assumptions by some scientists that these very components can be manufactured and produced by man and take the place of nature's food. All the while, these scientists ignore the body's ability or inability to digest and assimilate these processed and denatured products. It is the same as if they decided to use molecules of hydrogen and oxygen separately to water a plant. The plant will die being fed these disparate separated components. Of course, if it is given H20, water, the way nature presents it, the plant will flourish.

Nature cannot be surpassed

Let us remember there is NO confusion in the animal world about what to eat. There are no animals in nature weighing their food or concerning themselves about whether or not they are getting enough protein. There are no animals in nature taking supplements or concerning themselves about their calcium intake. There are no animals in nature eating according to their blood type. These concerns do not exist simply because these animals are abiding by the Laws of Nature and do not eat according to some institutional guideline, fashionable habit, or for the sake of entertainment.

Indigenous tribes dating back to antiquity have NO history of plague or chronic illness. These uncivilized tribal people did not experience obesity, heart dis-ease, cancer, "flu season," and the "normal" gamut of pains and infirmities our so-called civilized world suffers from every day. For example, the Native Americans were an incredibly fit and austere people, highly athletic, and robust. They had a deep reverence for nature of which they felt a part and they honored the Earth and the Sun. Then, the Mayflower arrived. This boat was filled with people who insisted, as our entire culture does today, that man was made to dominate and rule the world with ideas thought up by man that they insisted came from God.

The new foods, all highly refined by human genius, were introduced, including coffee, tea, alcohol, salt, and refined sugar. By the end of the 18th-century regular trade was established between the settlers and certain tribes. The new foods were consumed as well as alcohol, referred to as "fire water," and the new dis-eases appeared amongst the Native Americans. As the years rolled on, the Native Americans were perpetually brutalized and pushed off their lands by rapacious industrialists and the armies they commanded. These once fit and austere people were forced onto reservations, and as they continued to take on the "ways of the white-man" their health took a rapid and insidious turn for the worse. Centuries later, these once dynamic and spirited people on the Standard American Diet (S.A.D.) suffer all the indignities and debilitations that our infirm "modern" society endures.

The same example exists for many of the indigenous people of Central America, Caribbean Islands, Hawaiian

Islands, and Alaska where health and fitness was the rule until the refined, fried, degenerate foods and drinks were introduced. This phenomenon is already noticeable in Japan and is beginning to invade China, two countries where obesity was scarcely heard of. There is an obvious and undeniable link between the adulterated diet and dis-ease. The more "Americanized" or "modernized" these people become, the fatter and sicker they get.

Our national park rangers have turned into food police, doing their best to keep human food away from the wildlife, as these products create severe and immediate addictions in the animals who ingest them. Bears will literally rip doors off the cars that contain these heavily processed, sugared, and salted foods. These animals behave with a violent desperation, driven mad by their unnatural cravings brought on by exposure to these denatured and artificial foodstuffs. One would think if these products cause such bizarre and violent behavior in animals maybe this is not something we should be eating.

Anyone who saw the recent testimony of the tobacco company representatives swearing to a congressional committee that the use of tobacco and nicotine was harmless and not addictive will never forget just how willing men are to lie for a dollar. Who did they think they were kidding? Any human being with some sense can easily see the results of tobacco products and the strong addictions they create. No laboratory or scientists are necessary.

Is there any doubt that the soft drinks, candies, breakfast cereals, snacks, etc., that we eat and feed our children, are addictive and incredibly toxic? Rotting teeth and creating millions upon millions of stomach and skin disorders, these foods are packed with artificial flavors, colors, preservatives, and substances no human body was meant to digest. It is the responsibility of every adult to question what goes into their bodies and for parents to seriously inquire what they give their children to eat.

Living in accordance with nature's laws makes sense.

AS ABOVE, SO BELOW an ancient philosophical precept that is timeless and precise. Many great minds such as Plato and Pythagoras studied the similarities between man and the cosmos, the outer world vs. the inner world. In the past fifty or sixty years, quantum physics has had a tremendous impact on the way we view the universe. Recognizing the relationship between the micro-cosmos and the macro-cosmos is an invaluable key to understanding ourselves and the universe we live in. The study of our natural world may provide some needed guidance on the issue of nutrition.

The Earth is covered by over 70% water. The human body is made up of over 70% water. Whether animal or plant life, most organic life on Earth has a majority percentage of "organized water" as flesh. *Many of our fruits, all filled with mostly water as well; oranges, apples, avocados, mangos, lemons, tomatoes, grapefruits, melons, etc.* Given the fact that we are made up of mostly water, perhaps it would make sense to eat the foods that are also mostly water.

Notice the difference in texture and appearance of the flesh of a baby and that of an elderly person. You can feel and almost see the amount of water the baby's flesh carries and the obvious dryness and brittle qualities of the elderly flesh. This frail bodily condition of the elderly is not simply the result of the time spent on this planet, but the result of years of enduring a cooked, devitalized, toxic diet and many daily poisoning acts.

The more water-rich (percentage of water a food contains) a food is, the easier it is to digest. For instance, if you were to eat a piece of watermelon on an empty stomach, your body would be able to digest and assimilate that within a few minutes. However, any processed food from a piece of bread to a candy bar will take hours to digest, and although your body may feel a stimulating effect, the ingestion of this condensed food will place an unnecessary and unnatural strain on the body. This is known as enervation, a depletion of the body's nerve energy. We need to understand that:

Digestion takes a tremendous amount of energy.

If you need any practical evidence, think back to your last big gathering that involved a big American meat and potatoes meal. Think of the energy in the room before the meal. The noise and clamor make communication quite difficult.

As the meal begins, there is plenty of vociferous conversation, and getting somebody to pass the potatoes requires hand signals. As the meal goes on, the volume of voices and the amount of conversation begins to diminish. By the end of the meal, forks hitting the plate are easy to hear, and people begin to slump in their chairs, there really is not much to discuss anymore. The eating continues, and furtively, under the table, pants are loosened and unbuckled. The announcement is made that "dessert will be served in the den." Uncle Ted is nudged awake as you wonder if you can get to the next room without having to re-buckle your pants. The overstuffed reluctantly arise, calculating the shortest path to the most comfortable chair while calling out, "I'll have the apple pie." Positioning yourself in front of the couch you turn around and calculate the distance between you and the cushions, bend your knees and begin your descent that maybe just a little out of control.

You've landed safely, and soon the pie will arrive. You wonder how you're going to "get that pie down" but take comfort in the fact that you will not have to move for at least another hour and a half. Thank God for the TV, as talking is too much to ask for. Exhaustion has taken over. At least one or two are now out cold, and usually, one is comically snoring while others excuse themselves to find empty beds and couches to do some serious sleeping. It will take at least a few cups of coffee for anyone required to drive home.

This comical and quite familiar scene reveals the fact that digestion takes a large amount of energy. Of course, digesting a mass of cooked condensed foods and animal products puts a major strain on the digestive system. What are the repercussions of these daily unnatural feedings? They are many and quite severe. In fact, it is safe to say that at least 95% of our health problems are caused by the deranged and harmful feeding practices that have become part of our daily lives.

Fat

Obesity, one of this country's most severe health problems and a precursor to heart dis-ease, is caused by putting things into the body that cannot be digested or broken down. The way we get fat is by simply asking too much of our body's digestive capabilities and putting things into our body (in quality and quantity) that cannot be digested. When the body does not have the ability to digest these foods, the body will store what is undigested as fat. In its intelligence, the body stores the fat as far away from the vital organs as possible in the thighs, belly, chin, back of the arms, etc. As the poor feeding habits continue, the vital organs are eventually affected, the heart valves occlude, and acute dis-ease sets in. It is a tremendous strain for the body to pump blood through this inactive tissue (fat), and the added burden to the heart is evident.

It is a ludicrous and deceptive idea that "low-fat" foods like cheese, ice-cream, milk, bacon, bologna, ham, cereals, cookies, yogurt, bread, etc., all of which are heavily processed, will help in the efforts to lose weight. This premise of eating "low-fat" foods to lose weight is indicative of the confusion and misinformation promoted and extolled by our "experts," and another frightful example of the advice given by doctors and nutritionists.

If you want to lose weight and/or improve your health, your only concern ought to be the DIGESTIBILITY of the foods you eat, NOT the calories or the fat content. The word calorie comes from the word Kilocalorie, which is simply a unit of energy, nothing more or less. Counting calories is not nearly as important as asking the question "is this meant to be put in a human body?" If you are serious about losing weight and not gaining it back, this is the first question you will ask yourself before eating anything.

As far as fat goes, there are primarily four different kinds of fat: These include saturated fats, trans fats. monounsaturated fats and polyunsaturated fats. The lack of distinction between these different types of fat amongst our dieticians and doctors is a flagrant example of misleading information and abounding ignorance. Talking about fat reduction in the diet without recognizing these essential differences is ludicrous and another example of the thoughtless "science" that is pedaled on a daily basis.

The only fat that belongs in your body is unsaturated or polyunsaturated fat as is found in such foods as avocados, nuts, and seeds. This fat is easily digestible and utilized by the body as well as necessary for our wellbeing. Eating this type of fat DOES NOT cause you to be overweight. Saturated fats found in all animal products will make you fat, clog your arteries, thicken your blood, and wreak havoc on your digestive tract. Foods containing trans fat are even worse than saturated fats in that they contain hydrogenated oils. Liquids and oils

are turned to solids by combining this hydrogenated substance with the liquid. This creates something akin to
plastic bubbles, which are un-digestible and clog arteries as completely if not more than saturated fat. Once
again we find that our medical experts and nutritionists have long been promoting "low-fat" products such
as margarine and other hydrogenated foods as tools to
"lose weight and reduce the risk of heart disease." These
products do the exact opposite, as is evidenced by the
ever-increasing occurrence of heart disease and obesity. It
is worth mentioning that there is no such thing as being
"fat and healthy." No matter what agenda the media may
be promoting, it is a Lie.

It is nearly impossible to be a raw foodist and be
overweight.

Oils

You do not find oil, canned or bottled in nature. Many
companies swear by the use of the specific oil they may
be pedaling and all the health benefits they suggest will
be reaped. Flaxseed oil has been held up as a tonic that
carries great benefits and will help those who drink it
to overcome certain symptoms. The problem is that oils
of flax seeds, olives, peanuts, and almonds belong to
their respective seed or fruit. When extracted, oxygen-
ation immediately begins to set in and the oils begin to
decompose. MOST OF THE OILS WE BUY ARE
RANCID. Unless extracted, treated, and bottled with
great care, these oils have gone bad and are a burden to

our digestion. The very process to extract most oils is destructive to the product.

I once had the opportunity to taste some olive oil pressed in the Italian countryside. It looked quite different from the "extra virgin" oils I had seen before. It was a cloudy substance with a dense viscosity that tasted nothing like the oils I've had in the past. The point is the more processed a food (or oil in this case) is, the more difficult it is to digest.

By their lubricious nature, oils coat the digestive tract and interfere with proper absorption of nutrients and compromise the process of digestion. If you want to use olive oil, do your best to get the least processed oil you can find. The oil should be held in a very dark bottle and stored in a cool place and, like ANY food that does not occur in nature, used sparingly.

Dried fruit

Dried fruit, by its chewy and sweet nature, is a favorite food amongst those who are making the transition from the S.A.D. diet to raw foodism. It is a raw food with enzymes intact, however, it has been altered from its original state. Dried fruits obviously have less water in them, and the texture and sugar concentration has undergone significant changes in the drying process. These foods ought to be eaten in moderation as they can create toothaches and the urge to overeat. They also will take much longer to digest than fresh fruit and should be eaten alone.

Any sulfured dried fruit should be avoided entirely as sulfur is a known toxin. Be sure to ask your store manager or supplier if your dried fruit contains this deadly preservative.

You also may want to try soaking the dried fruit for a couple of hours. This re-hydration process makes the food much easier to chew and digest without losing any of the sweetness.

Remember the body is always doing it's best to repair itself and rid itself of poisons, but average Americans poison themselves forty to fifty times a day! Not only do we put such a poor quality of food in our bodies, but the quantity alone is absurd. The idea that we need to eat three meals a day plus snacks is a foolish and unfounded idea that in and of itself causes endless disease. When was the last time you saw a man or a woman live to be seventy or eighty who was more than thirty pounds over-weight? You do not see this very often simply because the body cannot maintain its life force carrying this added strain. There is only so much the human body can endure before it breaks down.

So if digestion takes all this energy, and our bodies need energy to detoxify, repair, and maintain themselves, it would make great sense NOT to put unnecessary burdens on our digestive system. We must do our best to "stay out of the way" and allow our bodies to do what needs to be done and this realization brings us to the biggest question . . . .

What is the best way to feed ourselves?

If you were out in the wilderness with no restaurants or fast food chains in sight and no refrigerators or "energy" bars in sight, sitting in an orange grove surrounded by wildlife and found yourself hungry, what do you think you would do to satisfy your hunger? Perhaps this is an unfair question and involves speculation for most of us, as few of us are ever in such a natural setting. Nonetheless, would you stare at the rabbits and deer and start drooling, wishing you had the speed to catch them? Would you charge after an animal in hopes of making a kill? Or would you put to use the best instrument ever made for picking and peeling fruits, the human hand? Go ahead, take a good look at your hand, open and close it a few times, check out how well your arm reaches over your head, and notice how well your nails are designed for peeling. What a natural instinct it is for us to want to climb trees, and how well designed we are for that activity. I'm guessing you'd pick the fruit and not assault any wildlife.

Having this wonderfully fragrant, beautifully colored sphere in your grasp would you begin to peel it and relish its sweet juicy taste, or would you begin to gather some wood and take the time to rub two sticks together long enough to start a fire so you could cook it? These questions obviously do not need answering but nonetheless need to be posed to see our bizarre behavior in a different light.

"Under souls rule, prince right-eating governs the gustatory estate. Guided by natural attraction. He supplies the right foods possessing all the necessary elements, especially fresh raw fruits and vegetables with natural flavors and undestroyed vitamins."

≈✦ BHAGAVAD GITA

There are over three hundred varieties of fruit of different sizes, shapes, and colors all with distinct flavors and nuances, ranging from our common fruits of apples, oranges, and bananas to the exotic varieties of durian, jackfruit, and cherimoya. Botanically speaking, any seed bearing plant food is classified as a fruit. Cucumbers, tomatoes, peppers, and sometimes avocados, usually referred to as vegetables, are in fact fruits. There is tantamount and clear evidence that the human body is set up for and will thrive on a fruitarian diet. There is no clearer evidence than your own experience.

Eating green leafy vegetables including celery, spinach, lettuce, etc., has become a point of contention amongst certain raw food proponents. Some claim this practice is unnecessary, and others claim it to be vital, while still others will say that vegetables ought to be eaten exclusively. After thirty years of study, investigation, and experience with myself and others, I have yet to see anyone become ill or suffer ANY detriment to their health from eating raw vegetables. I have noticed that eating raw broccoli or cauliflower can be a little difficult to digest. I have never had difficulty digesting any fruit. My desire and attraction towards fruit seem so natural, and the physical condition of my body and overall health is evidence enough to me that this is the way to go.

There is no doubt that human beings were designed to eat raw plant life. My impression is that eating mostly fruits is the best way to physically nourish our bodies. If you feel like eating raw vegetables, I can see no reason why you should not and would advise that the majority of your intake is fruit. I enjoy a fresh spinach salad, broccoli, vegetable juices and corn every once in a while and have been known to nibble on a carrot or two.

There is some plant food that you may want to avoid or eat sparingly. The simplest way to discern which foods these are is by asking a simple question. Would I eat this food for a meal? For instance, would you sit down and eat nothing but oranges for a meal? Obviously, there is no problem with that or with dining on melons, apples, mangos, bananas or pears. Would you sit down to eat nothing but (raw) onions for lunch? Not likely. How about a plate full of raw garlic? It would be less than a pleasant experience and perhaps quite painful This is the best way to decide what constitutes a whole food and what you should leave alone. Onions, garlic, and scallions all contain mustard oil, which is irritating to the digestive system and simply cannot be utilized by the body. These are irritants which ought to be avoided or used sparingly.

I know that there are many people who claim that garlic has some type of healing or cleansing quality. There is no doubt that ingesting garlic will cause the body to go into an immediate or emergency mode of elimination. To claim that the garlic is "helping" to cleanse the body as the body is being irritated and enervated by the garlic itself. You are just creating more problems. A healthy vital body will convulse at the first taste of raw garlic. The question I always put forth to those proponents of garlic, ginger, or any other herbal treatments is, "What is the cause of the symptoms you are trying to treat?" The next question is "Why not just remove the cause?"

Cooking destroys food. Incinerating your food will obviously render your food useless and completely devoid of nutrition, and you would soon die if forced to eat nothing but the black ashes of food remains. Just as heavy smoke can, within a few minutes, kill an individual forced to inhale it, we also know that smaller doses of smoke over time can also kill. Those who care about their health and their children's health keep themselves and their children clear of smoke as much as possible. There are many new laws being passed to protect the rights of those who wish to keep their lungs clean to protect from them from this obvious health hazard. Maybe someday we will realize the health predicaments that cooked foods create. We certainly would not feed our children ashes, just as we would not give them cigarettes. Why would we feed them (or ourselves) cooked foods? Pythagoras and the Pythagoreans understood the benefits of eating "unfired" foods. As his biographer informs us:

> . . . *the real reason, that he prohibited the eating of our fellow ensouled beings was that he wanted to accustom people to a contented life so that they should eat unfired (apura) food and drink plain water. Hence, they would have sharp minds and healthy bodies."*

—Diogenes Laertius, VIII 12

All cooked food is toxic.

If you were to take a cooked seed and plant it, it would not grow. The life-force has been destroyed. A tiny acorn the size of your thumbnail can grow into one of the mightiest trees on Earth because it has this magnificent life force present within it's being. Cooking destroys this awesome life force.

Have you noticed how difficult it is to remove the remnants of a cooked meal off a pot or a pan? How we literally need steel pads, various brushes, extremely hot water, and toxic chemicals to cut through the greasy and rock-hard food stuff. The cooked food has a cement-like stickiness to it that is no less sticky in your body. How difficult do you think it is for the body to deal with such a decomposed, devitalized, and denatured product? A bowl used to hold a fruit-salad can be effectively cleaned with a gentle rinse with no "elbow grease," no brushes or steel pads, no scrubbing, or cleaning agents required.

Putting cooked foods into a human body is biologically unsound.

Enzymes

The human body is not designed to digest dead, devitalized food, and the ingestion of such food stuffs is a great burden to the system and creates mucus and an acid, dis-eased condition in the body. When food is cooked above 130 degrees, ALL the enzymes in that food are destroyed. The destruction of these enzymes begins at approximately 104 degrees. Note that there is not much plant life in the desert where temperatures often reach 120 degrees and higher.

Enzymes are an essential to our well being. They conduct their force through protein molecules and are needed for almost every bodily function. A depletion of these enzymes wreaks havoc on all metabolic, digestive, and assimilative functions, and a body devoid of these enzymes will soon perish. There are four categories of enzymes. Amylase breaks down starch; Cellulase breaks down cellulose; Lipase breaks down fat; Protease is responsible for the breakdown of protein. The enzymatic content of a newborn baby is great, while the opposite is true for the commonly sick, elderly men and women of our generation. The reason that high fevers are so dangerous is that enzymes begin to be destroyed at a body temperature of 104 degrees.

Endogenous and exogenous enzymes include those that occur inside the body and those we get from outside (our food). If our diet is devoid of live enzymes, our body is forced to over-utilize its own reserves taxing the pancreas and intestines to supply more enzymes than they were designed to produce. Of course, the opposite is true. Eating a diet full of live enzymes creates the ideal situation in which our body's ability to repair and sustain itself is greatly enhanced.

A diet devoid of live enzymes is devastating to our glandular system that is responsible for regulating everything from our blood sugar to our appetite. The thyroid, pituitary, and pancreas are thrown into turmoil by an enzyme deficient diet, and this is the cause of many diseases from hypoglycemia to diabetes.

Closest to the vine is divine

ANY type of processing devitalizes live food. Cut an apple and watch how within a minute or two it begins the decomposing process known as oxidation and begins to turn brown. I am not suggesting you throw away all your knives and food processors I am just making the point that the less processed a food is, the better it is for you. If you have ever had the pleasure of eating a ripened fruit freshly picked off the vine, you already know what I'm talking about.

It is imperative that fruits (any seed bearing plant food, including avocados, cucumbers, tomatoes) be eaten on an empty stomach. The reason is that fruit does not digest in the stomach. It quickly passes through the stomach to digest in the small intestines. If there is a mass of cooked food struggling to digest in the stomach, the fruit will be trapped and end up rotting and putrefying, causing more problems. EAT FRUIT ON AN EMPTY STOMACH. There are many people that claim fruit does not agree with them, and they get upset stomachs when they do eat it. This stems from eating the fruit improperly.

It's also nature's requisite that you EAT YOUR FRUIT ONLY WHEN IT IS RIPE AND NOT WHEN IT IS TOO RIPE. Un-ripened fruit will stay acid in the body and can burn the stomach lining, whereas ripe fruit becomes alkaline when mixed with the enzyme ptyalin that is extant in the saliva. If your fruit is too ripe and fermenting, you will smell a hint of alcohol, this means the fruit is decomposing, overripe, and should not be eaten. Our bodies have NO use for fermentation or alcohol and must use vital energy to expurgate the foul substance.

It takes on an average of anywhere from three to eight hours (depending on what was ingested) for the body to digest cooked meals. If you want to make sure you are eating your fruit on an empty stomach, it may be wise to do so in the morning after your body has had at least eight hours of fasting. It is a good idea to see how long you can go into your day without ingesting any cooked foods. You'll be surprised at how your body will respond to this change. Work your way up to an entire day, and you'll be on your way to transforming your life. Remember there's no faster, more convenient food than fruit.

Sugar confusion

There are many people who are concerned about the sugar content in fruit. Many who have been diagnosed with hypoglycemia and diabetes are especially concerned. First of all, *comparing the sugar in fruit, fructose, with the processed, refined, and cooked sugars found in most other foods is a testament to the ignorance and recklessness of the "professionals" who do not see the biological, scientific, and logical difference between the two.* Lumping (couldn't help that) refined sugar in with the naturally occurring unprocessed sugars as something to avoid is no different from telling people, "Don't drink water or antifreeze." They are two completely different entities.

Our brains run on glucose. The fructose in fresh fruits is turned into glucose upon entering the digestive system. Refined sugars wreak havoc on a human body, throwing the endocrine system into fits and causing unnatural swings in the body's insulin levels. These abominations create severe mood swings and make addicts out of most who ingest these refined sugars. Please do not confuse the two. Realize that *there is never a reason to avoid eating our naturally intended diet.* Can you imagine telling a gorilla, "You've got to avoid bananas?" or telling a giraffe "Stay away from the leaves, they're no good for you?"

Fruit is the only karma-less food on the planet where no killing is involved. In nature when a fruit has ripened, the food falls from the tree. The plant or tree is not injured, and the seeds of the fruit are spread by the humans and animals who eat this gift from the gods, securing a procreation of more fruit-bearing trees and plants. Quite a beautiful design. Even when the fruit is picked before ripening, the tree is not harmed, and the fruit continues to ripen and blossom.

It is a testament to Mother Nature's organizational skills that there are hundreds of different varieties of fruit at our disposal. There are all different types of shapes, colors, fragrances, textures, and flavors, an endless array of delicious, nutritious choices. I do not know anyone, no matter how sickly they are or how deranged and desensitized their taste buds may be, who does not like some kind of fruit.

Hypoglycemia and diabetes

The millions of people who have been corralled into believing that the imbalance of their blood sugar levels is some kind of mysterious condition caused by bad luck, genetics, or happenstance, are constantly warned about ingesting their intended natural diet, fruit.

There are now over fifty different symptoms used to diagnose someone as being hypoglycemic. The list of symptoms which includes "mood swings," "headaches that come and go" (are there any headaches that are permanent?), "general fatigue," "difficulty getting up in the morning," "lethargy," "difficulty concentrating." According to these symptoms, our entire population is hypoglycemic. Considering what the average American puts into their bodies on a daily basis there is no way to avoid these symptoms.

"Diagnosis is so fraught with the element of uncertainty that no reliance can be placed on it."

≋✶ JOHN TILDEN MD (DR. TILDEN PRACTICED MEDICINE FOR OVER FIFTY YEARS.)

The condition called "diabetes," like all other dis-ease, is caused by putting things into the body that do not belong there. Insulin is responsible for facilitating the movement of glucose to leave the blood and enter the cells. Insulin is also responsible for stimulating the liver and muscle cells to convert glucose into glycogen, which is a carbohydrate and the central storage reserve for utilizable sugar in the body. Whether "Type 1" or "Type 2," diabetes is an insulin imbalance caused by a highly processed, cooked food diet that ravages the pancreatic function. The insulin treatments, (which once included cow and pig hormones and now made synthetically) given to millions of Americans create what is known in medical parlance as the "latter stages of disease," including poor circulation which can lead to amputation, dangerously high cholesterol, sexual dysfunction, impaired vision or blindness.

This disease, like all disease, is caused by putting things into the body that simply do not belong there. *The normalcy of the body is restored by proper living, not by artificially inducing the body to "adjust" to the existing malefic conditions through injections of pharmaceutical hormones. "Recovery" is available for those who wish to recognize the law of cause and effect and change their ways. Of course, if your body has become dependent on a certain drug or hormone it would not be wise to just stop the drugging altogether. Take into consideration the intensity and duration of the drugging to which you have exposed yourself and do your best to abide by the Laws of Nature. Remember that a fit body and mind makes the transition from sick to healthy that much easier.*

Food combining

There is much confusion about proper food combining. In a world where we literally have thousands of food choices, it is no wonder this has become an issue.

The easiest, most effective and natural way to eat and digest your food is to eat one food at a time. You do not need to have any other evidence than your own experience. Here's an experiment for you: On an empty stomach, eat a certain type of fruit by itself. If you are

eating pears, go ahead and have two pears; if you feel like
living on the edge, why not a third? Notice your energy
level in the next five to thirty minutes, you will experience NO enervation whatsoever. For your next meal have
a fruit salad with all your favorite fruits. Mix them all
together and enjoy. When you are finished take some
time to observe how you feel. You may feel just fine. You
may feel a little full or slightly fatigued. Your appetite
may have increased. You may notice some slight indigestion, and you will be certain that eating one food at a time
is really the most efficient and effective way to eat. It is
nature's suggestion to eat one food at a time. It might not
be the most entertaining way to eat, but look at the mess
we have gotten into by eating for entertainment's sake.

Animals in nature have no food combining issues
simply because they only eat one food at a time. There are
no salad bars in the jungle. If eating a mixture of raw foods
is the worst dietary habit you have, and you are experiencing no health difficulties, you need not concern yourself. I
do suggest that you take great precaution not to overeat, as
mixing foods does increase one's appetite. Once you have
established your natural diet, it would make sense to accli-
mate yourself to eating at least a meal a day consisting of
only one food.

Unfounded fears

There are certain raw food proponents that are professing the shortsighted and ridiculous practice that
the body has daily requirements of a very specific

combination and array of certain foods and nutrients, and this requires all types of daily measurements, diagrams (geometric shapes are very popular) and "systems." This idea is absurd, illogical, and completely without foundation. Flying in the face of nature's simplicity, the salesmanship goes on. The message pronounces "Nature does not understand like I do, you need my system to be well." It really is an embarrassing testament to man's egotism and foolishness. This approach creates confusion, undue fear, panic, and worry in those who wish to improve their health.

Remember that there are many well-documented cases of human beings who have gone over a hundred days without eating (with access to water) and survived. There also have been reports of human beings that simply do not eat. Most of these reported "breatharians" are highly spiritual people and live very simple lives. Many of the true religions of antiquity required their devotees to do forty-day fasts, taking only water. The human body has extraordinary wisdom and capabilities if we just would stay out of the way. Our bodies store amino acids and nutrients and can easily go months without taking ANY food.

The idea that you need a certain daily combination of sugars, carbohydrates, fats, or starches is a lie. A clean and healthy body absorbs nutrients so efficiently that surviving on one type of fruit alone is more advantageous than partaking in the morass of poisons the average citizen absorbs at every meal. The human body has extraordinary wisdom and capabilities if we just would stay out of the way.

Do not be fooled. Your health does not depend so much on what goes into your body or how it goes into your body as it does on what DOES NOT go into your body. In other words, all we really need to do to return to health is STOP poisoning the body. That's it. There is no need for all this confusion. Health is simple.

Because fruit passes through the stomach and digests in the small intestines, you must EAT FRUIT ON AN EMPTY STOMACH. Also, you must eat fruit BY ITSELF with no cooked or processed foods.

If you are eating a cooked meal it would behoove you to take some measures to aid your body. You can start your meal with a good sized salad (or a vegetable juice) with plenty of greens to provide you with some exogenous enzymes to help break down the devitalized enzyme-negated food and to help satiate your appetite. It is also a good idea to eat no more than one cooked or condensed food at a sitting, as the mixing of cooked foods creates a greater strain on the digestive capacities of the body and has a tendency to increase one's appetite.

Salt

Sodium chloride, or table salt, is a deadly poison that creates an acid condition in the body. All salt is poisonous. Whether from the sea or from a mine, it matters not. Salt will dehydrate your body, strain your kidneys harden your arteries, make your blood pressure soar and is a serious irritant to your digestive tract. Salt is a main cause of lip and genital sores (Modern Medicine calls it "herpes") as the body does all it can to remove it quickly through the skin, the body's number one eliminative organ. Salt is a baneful and unfortunately ubiquitous ingredient in all processed foods. You should never add salt to your food and do your best to avoid it at all costs.

Nuts

Rich in protein of high biological value, the nut is packed with vitamins and minerals and quite savory to man's taste. Nuts are rich in starches and sugars and contain far more vitamins than any piece of meat. Nuts will digest in the stomach and should be eaten alone or perhaps with some salad or vegetables.

Obviously nuts are nowhere near as water-rich as raw fruits or vegetables. Remembering the fact that the more water-rich a food is the easier it is to digest, we know that seeds and nuts are the most difficult raw food to digest but still easier to digest than ANY cooked foods. I have noticed an increased amount of mucus when eating regular portions of nuts. I suggest eating them sparingly. The longer you go on a raw food regime, the less you will desire this type of condensed food. Make sure to take the time to chew this food well to aid digestion. Beware of the tendency to eat handfuls at a time and to swallow the nuts before they are properly chewed.

Some nuts are more nutritious than others. The pecan, almond, coconut, pine nut, Brazil nut, pistachio, and walnut are amongst the best, nutritionally speaking. Make sure not to eat the skin of almonds (you can buy them blanched) as the skin is an astringent and can sometimes be irritating to the stomach lining. Brazil nuts are quite oily and may be difficult to digest depending on your constitution.

Cashews are actually not a nut but a seed of the cashew apple. This seed, unlike any other, grows outside the fruit. The cashew cannot be eaten in its raw state because of the cardol and anacardic, two little-known acids that will burn the mouth. The skin must be removed, and the cashew must be lightly heated in order to eat it.

To increase the digestibility of nuts, try soaking them in water for a couple of hours.

Of course, all nuts should also be eaten raw, unsalted, and unprocessed. Cooked nuts are acidic and the cause of severe indigestion.

Juicing

Always keep in mind the idea CLOSEST TO THE VINE IS DIVINE and remember that any type of processing will reduce the food's value. However, juicing can provide a wonderful method of resting the digestive tract without fasting. The greatest juicer in the world is our mouth. Its ability, with the help of enzymes in the saliva, to break down and masticate our food, is the first and perhaps the most important stage of food digestion. Chewing your food properly and thoroughly is always a great aid to your body.

Because digestion takes such a large amount of energy, any type of repose or rest will save energy. This energy will be utilized by the body to detoxify and purge itself of poisons. Fresh juices take very little energy to digest, and many nutrients are easily absorbed by the body. It is important to drink the juice slowly and allow every sip to stay in the mouth for five to ten seconds to let the juice mix with the salivary enzymes. DO NOT guzzle your juice.

It is also important to drink your juice immediately after squeezing it, as the breakdown of the food begins as soon as it is extracted. Obviously, AVOID ALL PASTEURIZED JUICES as pasteurization (a cooking process) destroys food. Fresh fruit juice is acid in the glass, but as soon as it mixes with the enzyme ptyalin in your saliva, it immediately becomes alkaline. On the other hand ALL pasteurized juices STAY acid in the body, burn the stomach lining, and help to rot teeth. If you are trying to lose weight and drinking acid juices, you might want to consider the fact that ANY acid condition or ingredient will cause your body to retain water, causing bloating to offset the acidity.

All cooked foods are unnatural and a burden to the body causing mucus, phlegm, fermentation, acidosis, indigestion, and an endless array of digestive problems from constipation to chronic diarrhea. However, there are some cooked foods that are less harmful than others. Steamed vegetables are the best-cooked food as they still retain some of their water. For this reason, it is very important that you do not overcook them. After steamed vegetables, there is a big drop off in the digestibility of cooked foods. The less processed a food, the better it is. Tofu, often thought of as a "health food," is heavily processed and incredibly difficult to digest. Foods that have been refined such as white flour, honey, white rice, sugar, salt, and those with chemical additives and preservatives are flat out dangerous to your well being.

Many people ask if brown rice is a health food. The answer is no. However, eating brown rice is much better than eating white rice as brown rice is less processed, so at least there is a possibility of absorbing some nutrients. Cooked rice is an extremely sticky substance. So adhesive are its properties that overcooked rice was once used as glue for book bindings.

The road to heaven

We have already established, that digesting cooked foods is tremendously enervating to the body and takes away from the body's capacity to detoxify. Eating such an unnatural diet prevents the body from performing its necessary and proper functions. Conversely, eating according to the Laws of Nature will allow your body all the energy required to push out any poisons and useless wastes.

That means that your body's eliminative powers will increase as you eliminate the counterfeit foods. This increase in nerve energy may cause some acute elimination through the skin, digestive tract, and/or respiratory system. Allowing these eliminations to run their course is necessary and natural. Understanding that this dis-ease (see Chapter 4 on Disease) is literally the way the body restores itself will allow for a relaxed acceptance of this natural process instead of the usual reactive urge to suppress the symptom with some type of treatment. It is crucial to ALLOW these eliminations to reach completion with no interference.

There is a wonderful saying: "the road to heaven goes straight through hell." Certainly most people do not have to go through "hell," but everyone will experience this certain boost in eliminative power. It may be an outbreak on the skin, an upset stomach, or a series of headaches, nausea, or general fatigue. All of these symptoms are commonplace to those who are making the transition. It is important to rest while going through these eliminations and not to concern yourself about feeling bad or looking bad. You must realize that you are literally ridding yourself of your old body. It is a sort of shedding.

Of course, this physical transformation will not occur without some discipline and sacrifice. The laws of the universe dictate that you do not get something for nothing. One of the most difficult aspects of the transition from the S.A.D. (Standard American Diet) diet to nature's way is the sometimes irresistible aroma of cooked foods. Living in restaurant laden New York City, it is impossible to avoid these sometimes delectable and inviting smells. I have not given up my love for these olfactory delights, but I have come up with a simple and successful strategy to stay with the regime that keeps me feeling so well.

I recognized the mechanical response I had to taking a whiff of some inviting smell and like most creatures immediately wanting to eat the food that I was smelling. I then wondered if it was possible to enjoy the smell of these foods without craving or even wanting them? After all, I love the smell of flowers, but never once did the enjoyment of their fragrance make me want to eat them. So I made some determined efforts to no longer associate smells with the desire to eat. This took some effort, but it can be done.

I still love the smell of coffee, still go out of my way to walk down East Sixth Street (Indian restaurant row) to take in the fantastic wafts of cooked herbs and spices, and I'm not shy to stand in certain pizzerias ("I'm waiting for a friend," I tell the men behind the counter) to get a good portion of those wonderful nose pleasures. Then I head home to eat some fruit or a salad. You can teach yourself to simply enjoy the smell of foods like you enjoy the smell of flowers . . . just a little rewiring is necessary.

It is quite common that those who go 100% raw will lose weight VERY quickly. Good news for most, but sometimes alarming for those who are already thin. Most of the time the body will go below its normal body weight sometimes up to ten to twelve pounds before coming back up to its natural intended weight. To many, this may be quite alarming, but it is nothing to worry about. If keeping weight on is important to you, I suggest doing some vigorous weight training and or calisthenics to build muscle tissue.

Organic

The general public has been catching on to the extremely dangerous and toxic pesticides, fungicides, and fertilizers corporate farms have been using to spray their crops. Again, man insists on attempting to control nature, and all those who ingest these poisonous pesticides are paying a heavy price. Cancer, bone dis-ease, respiratory and neurological failure, and an entire list of other health problems have been caused by exposure to these deadly chemical agents. Once again man's ego has created a devastating problem by working against nature. Some of the richest farmland in the world has been and goes on being destroyed.

There is NO reason for these baneful practices to continue, as there are so many natural farming techniques that not only will preserve the soil but will grow a much more nutritious and tasty product. Organic fruits not only taste MUCH better, they are significantly more nutritious.

Every time you buy a product you are, in effect, voting. Organic produce may be a little more expensive than the poisoned produce, but what would you rather do, spend a little more money, or swallow some carcinogenic nerve gas? These days, all across the country, most supermarkets are carrying organic produce. If you live in a smaller town I suggest you organize a food co-op. Co-ops are often successful enough so you can actually pay less for organic produce than you spend for non-organic produce.

If everyone decided to buy nothing but organic produce, it would mean an end to the poisonous commercial farming practices.

This would translate into less expensive and readily available organic produce for all of us. Buy Organic. Support the People that support your health and the health of our planet.

You may not always be able to find the organic produce you are looking for and may have to eat the inorganic stuff. I would highly suggest that you avoid eating any inorganic grapes, apples, strawberries, pears, or any other fruits or vegetables where you are forced to eat the skin. Many of these sprays and pesticides are water resistant, and a good washing does not do the job. If you must eat inorganic produce, you would be better off eating those foods that have a peel or a thick skin, such as bananas, avocados, melon, oranges, etc.

The answer to the question:

What should I eat to attain and maintain my optimum health?

Eat nothing but raw, organic, untreated, unprocessed fruits and vegetables, seeds and nuts.

I know the feeling that is coming over many of you who are reading this. "Is that it?!" "There must be more to it!" "Isn't there some kind of chart I can follow?" "What about getting enough protein?" "How many 'carbs' should I be taking in?" "This just seems too simple." "How do I know that I'm getting enough nutrients?" "My doctor says I can't eat fruit."

Ask yourself as honestly as you can, do you really want to be healthy, or *do you just enjoy talking about it?* Do you find yourself repeating the lie so often repeated, "I've tried everything and nothing works?" Do you enjoy complaining? Do you like to spend a lot of time trying out every new system introduced? Does all this energy spent distract you and take attention away from what really needs to be addressed? Are you ready to sacrifice your tacit fondness for the confusion, conversations, and drama surrounding your health and nutrition?

Health is not complicated, you are.

Anyone who is fed up with the constant pendulum swings from health to sickness, fat to not-so-fat, and fed up with their physical discomfort will begin to realize that the pleasures and comforts of the sensory world are the cause of their problems and will be thrilled to understand that health is, in fact, a very simple subject. Those that do not believe they have the capacity to sacrifice their addictions will deny nature's instructions, make false statements, and continue to relive the same disappointing experiences, maybe gaining some temporary relief along the way only to experience an increased misery down the road.

For some people, the idea of giving up their present way of living does not seem possible. The insatiable sense of taste is in full command, and no matter how damaging the effects, the possibility of superseding this sense does not seem possible or, for that matter, in the least desirable. YOU CAN CHANGE.

What if you really do not know what it means to be healthy? Maybe your idea of healthy means simply not being sick, or maybe it means being physically fit (there are many professional athletes with dis-eased bodies). What if being really healthy provided you with a CONSTANT sense of gratification instead of just a few moments at meal-time? What if re-gaining your natural birthright, true health, turned out to be the most exciting, freeing event of your entire life? What if really being healthy allowed you to sleep one less hour a night AND provided you with increased energy and vitality?

That would give you back over fifteen days a year. What could you do with all that time and energy? What would it mean to you to add another ten to fifteen dis-ease free years on to your life?

What would it mean to have faith that there really is a better way to live? What if you decided right now that you are going to find out for yourself if it is true or not? What if you said, "For the next month of my life I am going to do my best to live according to Nature's Laws and see for myself?" Remember you can always go back to your old habits.

It matters little what your present beliefs and imagined capabilities are. You are a living miracle with capabilities unimagined. Do not buy into your past experiences or your present way of thinking and take them for reality. You can do better.

4

WHAT IS DIS-EASE?

The myths and confusion surrounding dis-ease are rampant and more than obvious to the discerning eye and ear. We continue to live and abide by dark-aged perceptions, diagnoses, and treatments. The illusion of contagion and cures is as fixed in the mind of our culture as the fact that milk is a healthy food that builds strong bones (see Chapter 2 "Dairy Products"). It is obvious by the ever-increasing amount of dis-ease and sickness in our culture that the present paradigm for dis-ease and its treatment is futile and dis-ease producing in itself and often fatal. We are in this mess because we accept things as they appear to be and do not make the necessary efforts to find out how they

The disease and deformity around us certify the infraction of natural, intellectual, and moral laws, and often violation on violation to breed such compound misery.

≈ EMERSON

Happy is he who has been able to learn the cause of things.

☰✷ VIRGIL

Pain is consequent upon violation of the laws of nature.

☰✷ HERBERT SHELTON

really are. Disease, or dis-ease, means just that, the body is not at ease.

The human body is THE most magnificent and glorious invention ever created. It is a self-sustaining machine, independent and perfectly equipped for life on Earth. Seventy-five trillion cells work in unison, all of these cells imbued with an unfathomable intelligence. Everything we need for our health and well being has been provided on our planet, including the proper temperature, the right mixture of gasses in our atmosphere, all the necessary food, plenty of sunshine, and more water than we could ever need. Along with that, we have been provided with natural instincts that are constantly working to keep us safe.

Are you thinking for yourself? Or do you allow certain institutions, authorities, habitual and comfortable practices, cultural influences, and beliefs of the day to decide what is right and wrong? Is it possible for us to think for ourselves while living in a world where belief systems run so deep into the fabric of our society and daily lives?

Things are not always as they seem.

Despite the exponential technological advancements of our present era our society is still steeped in a tremendous amount of illusion and lying on many issues. Most people can hear the words and understand the idea of living in illusion and see how it might apply to others, but very few are willing to investigate the fact that the way we presently view dis-ease is as absurd and illogical as ever. Our beliefs concerning health and care of the body are dark-aged, superstitious, unscientific, and deadly. The problem is we all "know" so much and have an iron-clad trust in our present day experts.

It is better to know and think one does not know, than to not know and think one does.

≋ LAO-TZU

Unfortunately, most of us do not know and yet act as if we do. How many of us ever question what we repeat so readily as if it were fact? Despite our confidence and comfort in our scientific community, many of today's beliefs concerning health, dis-ease, and nutrition have no validity. It is important to remember that the power of illusion is great and can be the source of tremendous deception. Repeating things that we have been told, the parrot brain syndrome, is the very thing needed to create "realities" that have nothing to do with the truth.

Remember this . . .

Truth and force have no relationship.

Force cannot act upon the truth. No matter how many people believe and repeat misinformation, it has no bearing on what is.

Our present-day beliefs concerning health and disease are so entrenched in our psyche that a different model is almost impossible to consider, but that is precisely what is quite necessary for those who no longer wish to be confused and afraid when dealing with health issues. Those who are willing to question what we've been told are significantly rewarded and freed from the misunderstandings and delusions so prevalent in today's world.

The following is a different way of viewing the workings of the human body that will provide anyone with the opportunity to see for themselves by experiment and/or reasonable deduction if all this is truthful and logical as well as safe and effective. I am not telling you to buy my product or even to take my word for it but to experiment and see for yourself. It is a wonderful opportunity to gain control of your health no matter what your present condition. Do your best to empty your mind of all the things you think you "know" about health and dis-ease. Make some room for some new ways of thinking and remember that miracles are born of change of perception.

The truth will set you free is not just a cliché but a wonderful fact that is quite applicable to our physical health. Ok here is a different take on Disease:

> The body is a detoxifying machine. Any matter that is no longer needed or necessary in the body is marked for expulsion and taken out through many different channels. It is a natural event for the body to discard what is no longer needed. The eliminative organs are many: The skin, digestive tract, lungs, lymph system, kidneys, liver, spleen, etc., are always doing their best to keep our bodies clean. Twenty-four hours a day, seven days a week, three hundred and sixty-five days a year, our bodies are responding to whatever conditions to which we are exposed.

Eliminating waste and poison is a primary and almost constant function of the human body.

The more vital a human body is, the greater is its ability to rid itself of poisons.

After years of daily poisoning, a body begins to lose eliminative ability and vitality thus, poisons ingested stay in the body for longer periods of time and sometimes just do not get eliminated at all causing serious illnesses, such as heart dis-ease, tumors, nervous system disorders, and various cancers. By the way, cancer, or mutated cells are present in just about everybody. In a healthy organism, white blood cells capture and destroy these mutated cells; however, in a highly toxic body, the rate of mutation is accelerated, and these abnormal cells increase their proliferation. I have seen and continue to see those diagnosed with cancer return their bodies to health by abiding by Nature's Laws.

Here is an analogy that might be helpful in understanding how the body works.

Imagine holding a fifty-pound barbell and preparing to press the barbell over your head. The barbell represents toxins that must leave the body the strength of your muscles represents your body's eliminative vitality. Your body has decided to eliminate some poison and has the needed energy to do so. You begin pushing, and the barbell rising represents a cough or a fever or some other symptom or bodily expulsion. The body is at work expelling poisons. This is good and necessary. Yet we have been taught that this necessary and vital act must be stopped.

A drug is then ingested as "treatment" for the symptom. This is the equivalent of slapping another twenty pounds on the barbell, as all drugs are poisonous and put a dramatic strain on the body. Most of the time your body's eliminative process will shut down upon the introduction of a new poison as it only has so much energy. When the body finds it necessary to do some major cleansing, it may take some larger doses of poisonous drugs and antibiotics to debilitate the body enough to stop the natural eliminative process. The body now uses its energy to deal with this newly introduced poison and abandons the eliminative, cleansing process, so the barbell drops back down to its starting point. This is easy to demonstrate as everybody has gone through this very experience whether you are aware of it or not.

Can you remember the last time you went more than five or six hours or longer without eating? You may start to get a headache, feel faint, lightheaded, dizzy, and sometimes even suffer nausea or a fever. Then you remember you have not eaten in a while, so you grab a sandwich or a candy bar, or a soda or a cup of coffee. Immediately you feel better and relief has set in. This is a prime example of the body's elimination process being interfered with and shutting down in order to run the digestive system. When sickness comes on, the urge to eat is nullified by the intelligence of the body. The body, in a state of elimination, will cease creating appetitive circumstances until the elimination is complete.

Every morning you have the experience of the body cleansing itself. You wake up in a groggy state with some light-headedness and maybe even dizziness. Your tongue, a common channel of elimination, is coated with, a thick white film, your eyes have discharged a crusty substance, and the urge to stay in bed must be overcome by a screaming alarm clock, a shower, a cup of coffee or some other stimulant.

The body needs nerve energy to get rid of poisons and keep itself clean. The problem is in today's world the body is constantly battling to keep up with the endless array of contaminates ingested. When no food is taken in for a certain length of time, the body gains energy and begins elimination. As the body begins its elimination during this non-digestion period, poisons are dumped from the cells into the bloodstream in concentrated amounts, resulting in the symptoms listed above.

Despite the fact that this sick feeling is uncomfortable, it is the body's way of cleaning itself out, a vital function for sustaining its health. If we were wise and it was convenient, we would allow these symptoms to continue without interference . . . back to the weights.

As a result of the added twenty pounds of weight (drugs), the barbell drops back down to its original position and must remain there until the body can attain the required energy to push up seventy pounds. The body's intuitive process of elimination ends, and the illusion is created that the drugs have "restored health." The fact is that the body is now carrying more poisons than before and less able to deal with them. This illusion of "drugs that cure" continues to lead us astray and is responsible for the madness and confusion we now live in concerning health and dis-ease.

A vital, healthy baby ingesting any poison, including cow's milk, formula, salted and sugared baby foods, etc., will throw up, if not immediately, within a few minutes. Throwing up and regurgitation requires a lot of energy and vitality. Sadly enough, "throwing up" has become a baby ritual of our culture along with colic, ear infections, fevers, and other unnecessary agonies the child suffers.

As the baby continues to be assaulted by these toxins, the vitality of the body continues to drop. Instead of regurgitation and vomiting, the next eliminative channel, requiring less of the body's energy, is called into action. Skin rashes and fevers show up as the skin does its best to pour out the poisons poured in. As time goes on, the poor child is "treated" with drugs and pharmaceuticals (which are really more poisons and toxins) and fed a list of foods to "keep up the child's strength." With such "treatment," vitality is brought to an even lower level as the body struggles to endure the influx of pollutants. As the years go on, the devitalized body's lymph system becomes overloaded (mumps), lungs are immersed in mucus (various coughs, asthma), and the skin breaks out in acute rashes (chicken pox, or more chronically, acne). Allergies, hypoglycemia, diabetes as well as many behavioral disorders are a common part of all of our lives these days, and all are avoidable and reconcilable.

In today's world, ALL of the body's desperate attempts to purge itself are met with more poisons and "treatments" until the body is inundated with all it can handle and stops eliminating for months, sometimes years, at a time. Then, as we grow older, the onset of acute and intense eliminative efforts of the body known as flu, colds, and fevers, and other painful scary events are foisted upon us. These desperate attempts by the body to expel these poisons are continually met with an offensive and debilitating drugging regime that may suppress the symptoms for a short while, creating the illusion that the drugs work.

The symptoms may periodically end after a few days of ingesting drugs, and relief from this elimination may end for a while, but not only do the intended poisons to be eliminated remain in the body, more toxins are added. So the illusion created is quite sinister. We feel better, but the body is in a worse condition, enervated and devitalized, unable to push out the accumulated poisons. Because of this suppression and the increase in toxicity, the body may be unable to do what it must. The patient may feel better, but more serious and intense afflictions are inevitable such as, severe headaches, arthritis, tumors, nervous system disorders, liver failure, kidney failure, skin dis-ease, sexual impotence, heart dis-ease, and cancer.

What many of us view as strength and the ability to tolerate certain bodily abuses, such as binge eating or drinking, smoking, or the ingestion of other toxins, is in fact evidence of a devitalized and weakened body. In fact, anyone who has been abiding by the Laws of Nature for a year or more would be made ill and would most likely vomit upon ingesting many of the foods our culture regularly indulges in.

Nobody enjoyed their first cigarette. It was a painful experience, and the lungs convulsed and coughed repeatedly to push the smoke out, the eyes burned, and light-headedness and slight to severe nausea set in. As this habit increased and addiction to the nicotine set in, the body's vitality dropped severely, and smoking became first tolerable, then "enjoyable," much like our eating habits.

I cannot think of a more useless and insane habit than smoking cigarettes. If someone were to hold you down and force smoke into your lungs you could have them arrested and charged with a crime. You could easily show study after study that proves smoking destroys your lungs and teeth and makes you smell bad. Most people who die in fires do not die of the fire itself but die of the smoke inhalation. Yet millions of people are willing to PAY a considerable amount of money to assault and destroy their own body with smoke inhalation. There is NO ONE that doesn't KNOW that smoking causes Cancer yet people STILL do it and PAY for it. There is NOTHING glamorous about smoking. Hollywood movies and their CONSTANT and ubiquitous promotion of this insane, cancer causing, killer-habit over the past decades, is no doubt, partially responsible for millions of young people picking up this habit.

How many times have we heard the phrase "unexpected death" in reference to individuals who were "never sick?" This means they had lost all eliminative power, and the body's disability to detoxify resulted in death. They appeared "healthy" because the body was too enervated to expel the accumulating toxins. The body can only handle so much poison and still operate. There comes a time where it is simply overwhelmed and loses its life force. Medical men often refer to this phenomenon as "heart attack."

To view dis-ease as the cure it is and to stop trying to end symptoms is the only way we have a chance to gain true health instead of living life treating symptom after symptom. Trying to stop dis-ease is like trying to stop a steam engine from giving off steam, it is senseless.

What would happen if you were to stick a potato in your car's muffler and try to drive around? The car would shut down within a minute or two. It is necessary that the wastes are removed from the engine as efficiently and as quickly as possible. When the release of this engine waste is stopped, the car can no longer operate. The vehicle is forced to deal with a substance that cannot be utilized and is poison to its mechanics. The waste must be eliminated. Engineers and auto-mechanics know the importance of allowing waste to leave the machine as efficiently as possible and so design and maintain cars to do just that, eliminate.

Here is an entirely new way to view what we call disease:

- Dis-ease is the way the body takes care of itself.
- Dis-ease is the body's way of eliminating and dealing with poisons.
- Dis-ease is the cure.
- Trying to stop the bodies eliminative process is dangerous.

Not only are these efforts to stop dis-ease dangerous, but they are a complete affront to the laws of physics, logic, mechanics, and nature itself. When the body is purging itself we need to stand aside and let this dis-ease in the body run its course. We need to allow the poisons to leave the body as quickly as the body decides, and stay out of the way. Of course, it would make great sense to assess just what it was we put into this machine that did not belong there, and end the poisoning.

Stop the poisoning!

Now we're getting somewhere. If you are constantly cold in your new home, would you spend time bundling up and wearing your coat at the dinner table and dressing your family in winter clothes while you lounged around the house? Would you be satisfied that you had the proper gloves and hats and cozy scarves to keep your body's temperature up? Perhaps you could get by, and you could let your friends know that they had to dress accordingly when they came to visit. Maybe for some people, this would be a "solution." Others might want to investigate to see if there's another alternative, something more practical that might allow you and your family much more comfort and freedom in your home.

There are thousands hacking at the branches of evil to the one who is hacking at the root.

≈✴ THOREAU

Would it not make more sense to find out the CAUSE of the chill that blows through your home? Would you not want to check the windows and doors to see if they are closing properly and making sure there is no unwanted air blowing through the cracks? Would you not want to see why your heating system is failing and to check the walls for proper insulation. Only a fool would neglect to get to the cause of this uncomfortable situation and would continue to spend his time constantly bundled up like an Eskimo in his own home.

One of the great thinkers of our time has a wonderful quote that speaks directly to our society's absurd and dangerous methods of dealing with the sick (see Thoreau quote).

Treating the symptoms of dis-ease is the bizarre practice in which our health experts are continually involved. Hacking away at the symptoms is mostly an absurd practice that creates more dis-ease in the body and distracts us away from the message our bodies are sending us.

There are no shortcuts to health, but there are many shortcuts to the grave.

Another confusing, threatening, and errant practice is creating all the new and different names we have for disease. There are only so many ways a body can eliminate, so many ways a body deals with poisoning, and only so many ways that symptoms manifest themselves in a poisoned body. Diseases are named according to what eliminative channel the body uses to expel toxins, the intensity, and duration of this expulsion, and/or the consequential effects of the toxins in a body unable to eliminate. There are no "new" symptoms or "new" dis-eases. Diseases are also often named after its supposed place of origin such as "Asian Flu," West Nile virus, Ebola virus etc.

There is only one cause of dis-ease. There is only one cure.

Plato wrote about the extensive jargon used by the physicians of antiquity to describe dis-ease. Through the dialogue between his teacher Socrates and the character Glaucon, Plato scoffs at this nonsense.

> SOCRATES: Men fill themselves with water
> and winds as if their bodies were a marsh,
> compelling the ingenious sons of Asclepius
> to find more names of diseases, such as
> flatulence and cattarh; is not this, too, a
> disgrace?
>
> GLAUCON: They do certainly give very strange
> and new fangled names to disease.
>
> —*The Republic*, Chapter III (405).

If Socrates and Plato were alive today to see the HUNDREDS of newfangled names our doctors have come up with for body eliminations, they would fall over.

The point is that ALL dis-ease is caused by something. If you want to get rid of dis-ease, get rid of the cause. Do not be fooled by the deceptive diagnostic nomenclature and the *"necessary"* treatments doctors prescribe to scare and frighten you. Understand that there are constant efforts by the medical machine to literally promote new, and old diseases to create fear and panic and send people by the thousands to "get tested" for whatever it is they are promoting. Most medical tests are illogical, inaccurate and some are actually dangerous. STAY HOME. Study the Laws of Nature and begin to abide by them, you will immediately see your body respond once you get out of its way and allow healing to take place instead of trying to gain health by ingesting and/or injecting poisons.

The opportunity of illness

Dis-ease can also be a wonderful eye-opening consciousness inducing event. There are a few individuals who choose to view their physical challenges or present illness as opportunities for self-growth. These heroic souls know that they are never given a problem or challenge without also being given the opportunity to overcome it. The courageous efforts and sacrifices endured to overcome certain situations do nothing but build character in the individual and aid that man or woman in his or her self-evolution. No matter what happens to us, we ALWAYS have a choice of how we respond.

With each adversity lies the seed of an equal or greater benefit.

Some of the most horrible experiences human beings have endured have turned out to be the very thing that gives their life meaning. They discover that the greater the challenge, the greater the opportunity. I have witnessed too many miraculous recoveries from all types of grave and "hopeless" conditions to believe there is ANY ailment, disease, or physical injury that the human spirit cannot overcome. This indomitable human spirit combined with the alliance of Nature's Laws is a powerful concoction.

Dis-ease is our body's way of telling us that a severe imbalance exists. It is a signal that we are living in disharmony and that we need to amend our ways. The idea that dis-ease is random or contagious is absurd, which leads us to our next chapter which discusses the myth of contagion.

There are many well-intentioned people who participate in "awareness" and /or fund raising campaigns to "find the cure." PLEASE STOP walking, running, speaking out and marching to "increase awareness." No matter what disease you are marching for you are only aiding in the brainwashing. You are NOT "increasing awareness." If you REALLY want to help people you will apply the principles of a natural diet and become an example of a Healthy Human being. THAT will actually INCREASE AWARENESS and actually help people, instead of assisting the medical/pharmaceutical machine ensnare more people in their heinous "treatments."

THE MYTH OF CONTAGION

Bacteria are germs; germs are bacteria, and they are one and the same. According to many anthropological experts, bacteria were the first form of life on our Earth. Bacteria are necessary for ALL life on Earth. Our bodies are constantly teeming with millions of bacteria from our digestive tract to our eyebrows. Without these microscopic organisms performing their necessary functions, life is not possible.

Germs are present in all dis-eased bodies, germs are present in all healthy bodies. When germs are visible in diseased bodies, doctors claim them to be the cause of dis-ease. When dis-ease persists despite heavy drugging, doctors claim that "resistant" strains of these germs have developed, thus ensuring a profiteering drug cartel for years to come. If the people believe that there are constantly "new" and "resistant" strains of dis-ease producing

*Gentleman,
ninety-nine out
of every hundred
medical facts
are medical lies;
and medical
doctrines are, for
the most part,
stark staring
nonsense.*

∾✲ PROFESSOR
     GREGORY, MD,

invaders, they will also believe in the need to battle them with the new drugs.

Germs have been shown to be pleomorphic, meaning they change physical characteristics according to their surroundings. Studies have shown that their size, shape, color, and behavior respond directly to their environment.

Most human beings in this civilized world have large amounts of undigested, rotting, and fermenting foods in their digestive tracts and have bodies inundated with foreign and poisonous debris, a dis-eased environment. The bacteria living in such an odious environment are sure to be affected by such corrupt surroundings. The germs proliferate, multiply, and feed on the waste materials, and of course, the waste they produce is toxic, as is the food they take in. However, they are not the cause of dis-ease.

If you saw a pile of garbage and many flies and vermin feeding on this pile, would you claim that the flies and rats brought this garbage? The flies and rats are present because the garbage is present, they are not the cause of the garbage. Certain germs or bacteria are thriving because of the filthy environment, but they certainly are not the CAUSE of the filth or the discomfort or the dis-ease that ensues. This fact is so easily and commonly proven by those who are suffering dis-ease and take the proper actions by eliminating the ingestion of all toxins and allowing the body to restore it's health and letting the dis-ease run its course with no interference. The result is always the same: Health is restored.

At the turn of the century, a German doctor named Robert Koch did extensive studies on "microztmas" or germs. At the same time, Louis Pasteur had been doing extensive research trying, unsuccessfully, to prove that these micro-organisms were, in fact, the cause of dis-ease by injecting animals with the so-called "disease producers." Pasteur's experiments failed miserably. Despite the adverse results of his experiments, he proved his theories by falsifying and contorting lab results to conform to his desired outcome, a "scientific" tradition that continues today. There are few men that have done more to set back the health of humanity than Pasteur supported by the 'experts' who continue to espouse and regard his rampant lies. Despite his admitted plagiarisms and fraud, Pasteur is still revered by our confused society as a hero of medicine.

Dr. Koch was more interested in finding out the truth than becoming a popular figure. He had great reservations about the idea that microztmas (germs, bacteria) could cause dis-ease. Koch did his own studies and concluded that there were certain Laws of Nature and logic which could not be overlooked. He authored a series of postulates that directly address(ed) the idea of these presumed causative

> *This plagiarist (Pasteur) was the most monumental charlatan whose existence is disclosed to us in the entire recorded history of medicine.*
>
> ⇒* DR M. R. LEVENSON

agents. If a germ were to be declared "the cause of dis-ease," it would have to hold up to the following criteria.

The supposed disease causing germs must be:

- Found in every case of the disease.
- Never found apart from the disease.
- Capable of culture outside the body.
- Capable of producing by injection the same dis-ease as that undergone by the body from which they were taken.

These sensible, logical precepts were, and still are, revered by any true scientist or logical thinker although most doctors continue to overlook them, refusing to let the truth get in the way of their business. How can one claim that a certain and specific germ is the cause of dis-ease if it is not present in all cases of the disease? How does one claim causation if the germ is present but there is no disease? It is quite common to find those who have tuberculosis germs but no tuberculosis as well as those who have tuberculosis but no tuberculosis germs. The same goes for strep throat, pneumonia, the common cold, flu, and all the other so-called "germ-induced" diseases.

Doctors have conveniently come up with the notion of "susceptibility" to explain away the obvious incongruities of the germ theory. They claim that a weakened and debilitated body is in fact not dis-ease itself, but just a precursor to ill health and an invitation for the invisible microbe to "take over."

As the years have gone on, less and less often are germs (bacteria) claimed as the cause of dis-ease. In its place, modern medicine has touted the virus as a certain cause of dis-ease.

The virus myth

When Koch's Postulates destroyed the germ myth, the ever-expanding world of medicine and science needed a new culprit for the cause of dis-ease. A new enemy had to be found or created if they were going to continue to keep the populace in fear and sell their drugs. As the years went on and medical dominance grew, technological advancements provided a greater capacity for confusion and deception. The pressing need to find a real disease culprit, since the germ theory was incredible, was given a boost by technological advancement and the development of increasingly powerful microscopes. Modern medicine's second declaration of a disease causing entity was and remains far less credible than their original and, unbelievably, still believed germ fiasco.

Despite the fact that the word "virus" has become part of our daily lexicon, there are very few people who know anything about this entity. Our culture is once again caught up in the disastrous habit of repeating what we have been told and taking it for the truth. Stevie Wonder said it best, "When you believe in things that you don't understand, then you suffer, superstition ain't the way."

Over the years I have given lectures to thousands of people, and I often ask rooms full of people "How many people here actually know what a virus is?" This is always a poignant and revealing moment. It is rare that

ANYBODY raises his or her hand, and not once, among thousands of people, has one person been able to give an accurate description of this thing we so readily identify as "the cause of disease." The most common attempt to define a virus goes something like this, "I think it's a tiny germ that takes over a cell."

Wisdom is the recognition of our ignorance.

A virus is anywhere from one-one hundred thousandth to one billionth the size of a cell.
   A VIRUS DOES NOT:

- Ingest anything
- Leave any waste
- Propel itself in any way
- Reproduce on its own
- Show any sign of life

   A virus is inanimate, devoid of any type of capability to act in any manner.
   Doctors claim that a virus will "attach itself" to a cell or "inject itself" and then "command the cell to produce more virus until the cell explodes and spreads the virus to other cells." If this were the case, the exponential effect and chain reaction would cause every cell to be overtaken in a very short period of time. That never happens. Is it or is it not odd that our scientists would have us believe that our infinitely intelligent cells would "produce" their natural enemy? Nowhere else in nature does such an

abomination occur. Is there ONE example in nature of ANY species reproducing another species let alone its natural enemy? Ever hear of a mouse producing a cat or an antelope producing a lion?

There is no virologist in the world that can prove that a virus is capable of taking ANY action. If I asked you to believe that a piece of lifeless debris, one one-hundred-thousandth to one billionth the size of my body, maybe like a very tiny grain of sand, "attached itself" to me and then "took over" my body and caused serious illness, you might realize that sounds a little more than absurd. Imagine an elephant being "taken over" by a flea, a dead flea, and then the dead flea "commands" the elephant to produce more fleas until the elephant explodes.

Besides Modern Medicine's claims that viruses "inject themselves into cells and take them over," Modern Medicine also endows this lifeless entity with other superman-like qualities asserting that certain viruses are "tricky," "slow," "crafty," "smart," and they can "hideout," "lie dormant," and "gain dominance." If I told you that my chair mugged me, you would think I'm losing my mind. Inanimate objects, by definition, cannot act.

All cells have up to 30,000 tiny little organelles within their structure called mitochondria. Inside each of these little organisms (mitochondria) lies a piece of DNA (deoxyribonucleic acid) that is encased in a protein shell. On average we lose about 500,000,000 cells per day. There is an enzyme producing organelle called a lysosome that helps to break down these dead cells and prepare them for elimination. Other cells commonly use the debris of the dead cells for their own sustenance and through the process of phagocytosis take in parts of the cell, and the rest of the dead cell gets eliminated through the many different channels our bodies use to cleanse itself. What our doctors and scientists refer to as a "virus" is simply this protein encased piece of DNA, It is cellular debris in various stages of decomposition. A *"virus"* is indigenous, organic, lifeless, waste material.

By closing the eyes and slumbering and consenting to be deceived by shows, men establish and confirm their daily life of routine and habit everywhere, which still is built on purely illusory foundations.

≋✲ THOREAU

What a tragedy that we have bought into such lunacy and never take the time to question what we have been told. Our society is enslaved by this abounding ignorance. We are relegated to abiding in bizarre, unnatural, dis-ease producing, and often deadly drugging regimes in the effort to maintain or regain our health, depending on a "science" based in delusion, all because we fail to verify what we have been told.

The grand illusion

The myth of contagion is one of medicine's chief foundations, and one of the public's favorite. Only those that lie to themselves will believe in lies. Lying to yourself includes being ill-informed or being ignorant or pretending that you "know" because you have heard something repeated so many times. Many people embrace the idea that they are not responsible for their health and that they are "susceptible" to the foreign invaders that take them over. The tendency we have in our emotional lives to blame others for our unhappiness and constantly to focus and place responsibility for our misery everywhere else but on ourselves is directly reflected in our culture's view of dis-ease.

It is a fascinating study to see how modern medicine chooses to name dis-eases such as "Russian Flu," "Beijing Flu" (post-Tiananmen Square), "German Measles" (if the Communists bugs don't get us, the Nazi bugs will). It is equally fascinating to notice where dis-eases supposedly originate; "Aids," as well as the Eboli virus and the "West Nile-like Flu," came from far away Africa. The subliminal messages are, "You are not responsible for your health because foreigners are, but don't worry we have drugs that will save you," and "your sickness has nothing to do with your obscene overeating and disregard for proper feeding." It is quite a comfortable situation to live recklessly with no consideration concerning food choices or lifestyle and have the luxury of blaming our illness on a foreign invader. This refusal to take responsibility for our health makes fertile ground for the seeds of deception. Most prefer the comfortable to the real.

Let us take a look at the present illusion of contagion that exists. It is a relevant inquiry and not only explainable but verifiable to all who endeavor to learn.

"If contagion does not exist, how do you explain the plague?" Good question.

The Black Plague that ravaged Europe's populace in medieval times appears to be a clear testament in favor of the theory of contagion. Medical experts to this day agree that the plague was spread by "fleas living on the backs of rats." There is another explanation much more feasible and closer to the truth. All dis-ease is caused by poisoning acts, there was no shortage of such behavior in the Dark Ages.

In many European towns and villages filled with the poor and destitute, a stiff tax was charged to those who wanted windows on their dwellings. The result was that many people, sometimes three generations worth, lived in one overcrowded dwelling devoid of sunlight and fresh air, two of our most health-giving natural gifts. It was common to sleep five or six to a bed in these unventilated dwellings. Horse manure was commonly used to stop up any opening where cold air might enter. Fireplaces sucked up the already small supply of air. Superstitions and fears abounded concerning demons, and the human body was looked upon as evil and was denigrated by those who were "godly" men and women. Bathing was not part of any daily regime, and nudity was shameful and scorned. Thus very few citizens ever bathed or allowed the sun on their skin, and physical hygiene was at an all-time low. Clothes were rarely if ever changed or washed. It was common for the world-renouncing fanatics of that age to welcome dis-ease as a sign of divine favor and to revel in physical decrepitude. Man tried to immortalize his spirit by maligning his flesh.

There were no sewer systems, and garbage and human waste were commonly dumped in the street, creating a disgusting and foul combination with which citizens were forced to live: So they covered their mouths and noses with thick cloth as they walked along to prevent gagging and nausea. It was common to let the garbage pile up until the narrow corridor-like streets had to be cleared so that horse and pedestrian traffic could resume.

The diet of the day was mostly animal products. Lard (animal fat) pies were common, as they were cheap and readily available. Eating fruits and vegetables was not so common because these foods were thought to be devoid of nutrition. Lead utensils were utilized, and sanitation in food preparation was nonexistent. Oftentimes the water supply consisted of a stagnant moat that surrounded the village; there was no running water.

Due to these filthy living conditions, lymph glands would swell, and the physicians of the day would treat this condition by a "good blood-letting" (which involved opening up a vein and draining large amounts of blood from the patient) or by surgically removing the glands (a common practice of today's modern medicine with tonsils that swell, "overactive" thyroid, or a women's breast "as a preventative measure" to avoid breast cancer). These operations and treatments done in filthy and primitive conditions obviously did nothing to improve anyone's condition and were the direct cause of many deaths.

ANY society living in this kind of filth and squalor would experience "plague," rat-back fleas or not.

The plague ended as entire villages and towns were burned down, many people moved to more rural settings, new architecture was erected, sewer systems were built, and the Renaissance brought with it the beginning of the end to backward thinking and an appreciation of humanity, which translated into improved sanitary and social conditions. There was no such thing as vaccines, and dis-ease disappeared as fast as the filthy living habits did.

There is no history of plagues from the years 800 BC to 400 AD. The Greeks and the Romans had created extraordinary civilizations that influenced all of western culture.

There were public baths in every large city, fresh water, and a large part of the diet was fresh fruits and vegetables. Athletics was a prominent part of the culture, and pride was taken in a fit and vigorous body. Dietetics and private and public hygiene were high on the list of these thriving cultures until gluttony, greed, and corruption befell them.

"What about family members, school children, or office workers that get sick in succession or all at once? Isn't that evidence of contagion?" It certainly appears as if this common occurrence is "evidence" that dis-ease is "caught." Upon closer review, another conclusion is verifiable.

Families living under the same roof are exposed to and partake in the same poisoning acts. These include the same water and air supply as well as the same foods, attitudes, and emotional stresses. By partaking in all these similar or identical activities the chances of similar and common poisonings and body-initiated purging (illness) amongst the family is great. Of course, some family members have more vitality than others, and the effects on each member will vary, causing some to, get sick immediately and others a few days later or not at all.

When is "flu season?" It usually starts at the end of November, and really hits home by January and February, directly following Thanksgiving, Christmas, Hanukkah, and the New Year. What kind of activities do we partake in? Let's see: There's increased drinking, emotional turmoil, financial burdens, plenty of gorging and overeating. Couple this with the fact that there is less sunshine in these winter months and less outdoor activity which translates into less fresh air and no sun on the skin plus the emotional dreariness and let downs of our high expectations for the holidays. The drop in temperature and freezing conditions add to the mix of taxing the body. There are also the inoculations of poisonous and sometimes deadly flu vaccines filled with mercury, aluminum, formaldehyde, and animal pus that our physicians inject us with as a "preventative measure" that add to this recipe for the illness that we call "flu season."

There is also the plain fact that there are tacit rewards for being sick. As a child who did not enjoy school, I knew if I could make myself sick, or at least appear to be sick, the reward was great. I got to stay home, watch TV, and get a lot more attention than I normally would. Looking back, I was often surprised that I would actually start to feel ill after acting the part for a certain duration, a testament to the power of thought.

There is so much power in belief.

Modern medicine is constantly proving the power of the mind by doing medical studies with placebos. It is quite common for people to get well, simply because of their faith in the bread or sugar pills that they are given which they believe are medicine. It is quite clear to any objective observer that people get well in spite of their treatments due to their strong beliefs.

Healers in certain indigenous tribes perform a ritual called "bone pointing." The tribe gathers around the healer who spins a bone. Whoever the bone ends up pointing at is believed to be doomed. Because of the strength of the belief, this individual may actually perish. Similarly, people under hypnosis may actually perceive a burning sensation when touching an ice cube after the suggestion that the ice is burning hot.

Is it possible that our civilized world can be viewed as a tribe also, and that we are under a sort of hypnosis? Could our own set of belief systems be so embedded in our psyche that we think ourselves sick? When the flu or virus of the season is so prominent in our daily discussions, could our unconscious belief in virus-caused illness itself create dis-ease, especially since there are rewards to be had?

Is there any doubt we would have fewer sick people if companies gave "health days" out to their employees instead of "sick days?" Employees in my company would be told that they are allowed ten days a year to take off to keep themselves healthy, and those that did so and stayed healthy for an entire year would receive a bonus. If companies took on this policy, without any change of diet, the number of sick employees immediately would be halved.

Maybe you know of a person who is constantly complaining and bitter? This person is bound to be a sickly individual and in constant physical turmoil. You may also know a person who is genuinely cheerful and optimistic and notice that this person is full of physical vitality and

THE MYTH OF CONTAGION

enthusiasm for life. Our beliefs and general attitudes are the most powerful factors in the creation of health or disease. (See Chapter 9)

As with any widespread superstitious belief, our tacit agreement with the germ and virus myth has our entire population living in tremendous fear and has kept the entire world populace unconsciously dependent on the products of the instigators of this deceptive myth. It is rare to find any American family without some type of pharmaceutical dependence, and it is just getting worse as the medical machine continues to promote and invent "new" disease and scare parents into drugging their children and babies as early as possible. "Start 'ern young and early," is no different from the strategies of the tobacco companies and their powerful marketing techniques to teenagers.

The medical notion of contagion is a hapless, wretched lie.

If you would like to see for yourself whether or not all of this is true, there is a very simple and scientific test you can conduct. Begin to study and abide by the Laws of Nature and let your body detoxify without interfering. Stop all poisoning acts, keep an exercise regime, feed your mind and heart with loving, life-affirming ideas, and you will experience the health you were intended to live with. You can then hang around all the flu-ridden friends and relatives you want, and you will not be affected. How can I be so sure? Because I have not had "the flu" in 30 years, and I am commonly in contact with those who are sickly. The same goes for the many people I know who eat according to their biology.

The idea that you could "catch" dis-ease is as absurd as the idea that you could "catch" health. Of course, exposing yourself to extreme cold or heat for significant periods of time could cause illness and eventually death.

Here is a wonderful invitation to rid yourself of the idea that dis-ease of the body is contagious. You've got nothing to lose but your fear and dis-ease.

CHAPTER

6

FASTING

When animals in nature are sick or injured, they have a natural instinct to abstain from food. This inanition allows the body to utilize ALL its force for the healing required.

Even house pets who exist on the destructive cooked food diet have the instinct to avoid food until they are well. It is only we "civilized" human beings who insist on eating while sick in order to, ostensibly, "keep up our strength."

Despite the beliefs of the day, the quickest way to return a human body back to health is to completely allow the body to use all its nerve energy to purge and detoxify itself. This condition is achieved by the cessation of food intake and by drinking only enough water to satisfy thirst.

With the discontinuation of feeding, the body will utilize all the fat, bodily excesses, and un-metabolized food the overburdened digestive tract carries. After an extended period of digestive rest, the unnecessary, super-fluous, and toxic matter in the body is broken down, utilized, and expelled, leaving the body in a cleaner, revitalized state. I have repeatedly witnessed significant tumors shrink and disappear during prolonged fasts. A physical "rebirth," is how the results of an extended fast are often described.

In spite of the miraculous claims of certain "cleansing" products and "fasting techniques" there is no more purer, effective, or hygienic approach than a pure fast. The body does not need any help in doing what it knows best. Any kind of stimulant, be it an herb, cayenne pepper, psyllium husks, intestinal *cleansers*, or oils, is a hindrance to the ultimate goal of a clean body.

Along with the returned elasticity and clarity of skin, finer muscle tone, clearer eyes, and a sharper mind, the increase in energy and the ability to the assimilate food the way it was meant to be is dramatically heightened by fasting. A certain high is achieved that has nothing to do with stimulation and everything to do with feeling what it is like to live in a properly functioning, detoxified human body. Sadly, this is a state most human beings will never experience due to our constant gluttony and fear of going without food for more than a few hours.

Fasting is NOT starving. The human body uses glucose, complex sugars, and carbohydrates as its initial source of energy. When these sugars are burned up, the body will then begin to burn fat as its subsequent energy source. The last thing a body will use for energy is pro-tein. Most human bodies could easily go thirty or forty days before the body goes into the harmful state of using muscle tissue for its survival. This state of ketosis, the beginning of starvation, is the final attempt of the body to survive by literally digesting itself. There is so much bodily waste and fat tissue on civilized man that it would not be surprising if the average American could easily survive for much longer than forty days without food. Although the restorative and recuperative powers of a fast are evident and highly regarded by those who understand nature's ways, this rejuvenating effort is highly misunderstood and ignored by our present-day "health" officials. Most of the time it is only the desperately ill that look into nature's cure with any real consideration, as giving up eating is simply not high on the list of viable treatments when in fact it is THE quickest way to return one's health.

Great caution must be taken before engaging in a fast. Fasting will supply all the body's nerve energy to the eliminative organs. In a body that is highly toxic, this could mean danger. Although rare, it is possible for the eliminative organs, such as the kidneys, liver, or lungs, to be overworked, and possibly fail, if the concentration of toxins is too high.

To avoid any serious difficulty, it would make sense to clean your body out gradually for a long duration before beginning a prolonged fast of three or more days. Fat cells contain much more toxins than do muscle or bone cells, so losing weight and being close to, or at, your intended body weight is an ideal way to begin a fast, along with serious consideration of your past and the amount of poisons you have ingested or been exposed to. It is also highly recommended that you get yourself in the best physical condition you can before beginning a fast.

If you have a long history of drugging, whether illicit or prescribed, smoking, drinking or any other type of prolonged poisoning, DO NOT attempt an immediate fast unless you are in a very serious health crises. Without making fasting out to sound more perilous than it is, I have seen people embark on a fast completely unprepared for the journey with little or no understanding of what is to come and end up in a panic, desperate and confused.

If you fall into the category of a highly toxified individual, you can progressively work your way up to a pure fast. It would make sense to find someone who has experience and expertise in this area to assist you. Before any type of fasting, it would make sense to eliminate all poisons in your diet and begin a raw food regime. This will immediately begin to allow the body to start the long process of eliminating without any danger of detoxing too quickly. After establishing your new eating habits for a few weeks, you could invoke a short juice "fast," which involves taking nothing but fresh juices for one or two days at a time.

Any type of fast will initiate body eliminations of different degrees, which may include skin outbreaks, headaches, diarrhea, nausea, fevers, lethargy, or all of the above. It is very important to have an understanding of the effects of digestive rest (fast) and prepare yourself for the ensuing conditions that may follow.

Make sure that you allow yourself plenty of rest and keep your activities to a minimum. The idea behind fasting is to rest not just your digestive system but your entire body. You may have no choice as often times the effects of bodily purging will be physically exhausting. Some people however, may have bursts of energy that may last days and actually find it difficult to sleep for more than a few hours, every body is different. Your attitude and mental approach will play a MAJOR role in how difficult or easy a time you have. UNDERSTANDING how your body may respond and exactly just what is happening while you are fasting is imperative. One thing you can be assured of, your efforts will bring you closer each day to the miraculous state you were meant to abide in, that state, rarely experienced, is true HEALTH.

It is very common on a prolonged fast to have powerful urges toward certain foods. These addictive responses are brought on by cells releasing certain toxins into the bloodstream for elimination. This condition is responsible for bringing on such powerful urges or withdrawal symptoms. Cooked processed foods are extremely addicting. There is also the possibility that after the first day of fasting you literally will not be interested in food, this is always an unexpected and great help. As your body starts the process of purging itself, the release of appetitive and digestive enzymes will cease completely so that your interest in food is minimal or nonexistent.

"Fasting to completion," means that your body has been completely purged of toxins and waste. This could take anywhere from five to forty days depending how polluted your body is and how vital your eliminative organs are. You will know when you have fasted to completion by some unmistakable physiological signs.

As you are going through your fast, you may experience a thick white coat forming on the tongue, bad breath, loss of appetite, skin eruptions, and a dark discharge in the urine. When the body is completely cleaned, the tongue will become clear, the breath sweet, the eyes extremely clear, the appetite will return, the skin revitalized and the urine will become clear like water. These are the signs your body has completed the cleansing.

Obviously fasting to completion is a major effort that requires a set of circumstances that will allow you to get the proper rest and stay in bed for days at a time, perhaps even weeks, if you are highly toxic. You may have to break your fast before the body has completed its cleansing because of certain life demands.

Breaking the fast requires great caution. The longer the fast, the more caution is required. Tremendous damage can be done to the body by overfeeding after a prolonged fast. If you have gone for more than five days without food, it is highly recommended that you ingest only a small amount of fresh juice on your first day of eating. It is helpful to dilute the juice with water at first, as this will gently bring the body back to its digestive functions. Your first few meals must be extremely small and include one highly water-rich fruit, such as watermelon, oranges, or grapefruits. Do not mix any foods after a fast. Do not eat until you are full. Stick to a mono-diet (one food per meal) for at least two or three days. Absolutely no cooked food should be taken for AT LEAST one week following a fast and a minimal portion at that, if you must.

As you continue to adapt to your natural way of feeding, the body will become cleaner, more efficient, and will easily adapt to any fasting regime. For years, I have taken on the habit of taking at least one day a week to fast and rest my digestive system. This practice has completely changed my relationship with food. I used to think that food was necessary to keep my energy up. It is now quite clear to me that my energy level is at its peak when taking no food. I can do a vigorous workout for two hours, go through a full day without eating a thing, and feel incredibly energized. I need two hours less sleep on the days that I fast, and any mental exercise is completed with greater efficiency and adeptness.

It does not really make much sense to have the finest car in the world and never clean out the carburetor, change the oil, or replace the oil filter. This type of upkeep is expected and required to keep the machine running the way it was intended. Any sort of negligence towards the machine would noticeably be reflected in its performance. It is the same with a human machine, our bodies need tune-ups also. In fact, given the sorry state of our feeding practices, the man or woman existing on the "civilized" diet requires ten times the amount of care than any automobile. Fasting is a wonderful way to allow the body to tune itself up.

Many people claim that they just do not have the time to lose weight. IT DOES NOT TAKE ANY TIME TO NOT TO EAT.

CHAPTER

7

VITAMINS, HERBS, WATER, AND SUNSHINE

Despite our technological advancements, the body remains a mystery. There are no scientists who can even begin to explain the force that animates our cells and gives life to this organized accumulation of matter, the human body. We have learned a large amount in the past fifty years, but the present knowledge and understanding is still very limited at best. In the past fifty years, the number of recognizable vitamins in our food and those used by our bodies has tripled. As time goes on, more and more information is gathered and accumulated, and the new understandings often contradict the old ones. The expert advice of vitamin salesmen continues to change from year to year so that the expert advice of five years ago is now deemed obsolete. And the advice of today will be opposed by the same experts who are now so sure of themselves and dispensing that very advice.

As mentioned earlier in this book, it is common practice for our scientists and biochemists to pull apart and isolate certain nutrients in the foods we eat. Why is this being done? First of all very few people have any understanding of health or healthy practices, and our society LOVES the idea of a quick fix remedy to solve our problems. Second of all, most of our populace has been convinced or likes to believe that health can be restored by taking the proper pills. Add to the mix the health provider's realization that there are tens of millions of dollars to be made selling vitamins to a shortsighted public. You can bet that wherever and whenever health is lacking, Natural Laws are being ignored. THERE IS NO SUBSTITUTE FOR PROPER FEEDING. Just like there is no substitute for fresh air, exercise or sunshine.

The problem with any vitamin is that little or no consideration has been given to the conditions necessary for its proper assimilation into the body. It is quite clear that vitamins and minerals are absorbed and assimilated into the body in specific combinations. These natural combinations exist in perfect sequence and abundance in nature's fruits, vegetables, seeds, and nuts. To extract one element of a food, highly process it into some type of powder, and imagine its absorption capabilities will be unaffected by its separation, is the same thing as imaging you can make a phone call by dialing just one number or bake a cake with one ingredient. In addition, any life force is destroyed by the processing. Also, it is no secret that many of these vitamin products sit on the shelf for months and sometimes years at a time.

During certain famines, people have attempted to eat the soil in order to stay alive, with the hope that "since plants live off the soil, so maybe we can too." Desperate times call for desperate measures, but obviously, human beings or any other mammal cannot survive eating soil. We need the bio-logical synthesis of plants to absorb minerals from the earth and convert them into readily available organic nutrients our bodies can use. The plants' remarkable biological synthesis of minerals is not yet fully understood by our scientists and certainly cannot be reproduced in a laboratory.

Our bodies are made up of iron, phosphorus, iodine, copper, magnesium, etc., the same minerals that are also found in the soil. But the vitamins and minerals found in the soil are unusable in our bodies; they are inorganic minerals that must be synthesized by plants before being taken into a human body. Biochemists and vitamin companies refuse to recognize or admit the simple fact that INORGANIC (un-synthesized) MINERALS ARE UNUSABLE AND TOXIC IN THE BODY.

Even vitamins and minerals taken from organic sources including plants and animals are vitiated and made unusable by heavy processing and packaging. Many vitamin pills contain refined sugars, salts, gelatins, and artificial sweeteners. The result is that the body, instead of being fed and assisted, is toxified and enervated.

The biochemist looks on all dis-ease or symptoms as a lack of a certain element or elements, ignoring the fact that dis-ease is created by poisoning acts. Even in persons who do lack certain elements, the lack is created by some type of poisoning or unnatural feeding and certainly will not be resolved by ingesting the inorganic elements found in soil.

If you are concerned that you are not getting enough of a certain vitamin, you would be better off finding out what fruit, vegetable, seed, or nut is rich in that particular vitamin, and eat that instead of taking a pill. This way you can be sure that your body has the ability to absorb the nutrients the way nature intended. Remember that our bodies need so little food and that deficiencies only will occur if you refuse to recognize your biological set and defile the body with pharmaceuticals and/or poor grade foods and drinks.

I am happy to report that there are some vitamin manufacturers who understand these ideas and have products on the market that actually may help an individual who refuses to change their diet.

I would recommend to the many out there who will not give up their harmful ways to simply add a freshly squeezed vegetable or fruit juice on a daily basis to give your body a chance to take in some real nutrition.

What about herbs?

Echinacea, goldenseal, various roots, and many other herbs have gained tremendous popularity in the past ten years. I am thankful to see that there are millions of people recognizing the poisonous nature and deadly "side"-effects of the drugs the pharmaceutical companies continue to peddle. According to the Wall Street Journal, there are "128,000 deaths a year from improperly taken prescription drugs." I wonder how many deaths there are from properly taken prescription drugs?

It is great that people are looking to the alternative methods for the treatment of dis-ease. Despite all the hype over herbal remedies, the wise man or woman will realize that there really is no shortcut or alternative to healthy living.

The essential message of this book is that ALL dis-ease is caused by something, and the only real solution is to get to the root of the problem and eliminate it. *If there is no cause of dis-ease, there will be no symptoms of dis-ease.* Herbs are given as remedies to alleviate certain symptoms. They have a stimulating effect on the body and cause certain organs to go into a state of rapid elimination due to the irritation the herbs cause. This is quite enervating to the body and each time an organ is artificially stimulated or poisoned, it loses some of its inherent efficacy. There is no such thing as a free lunch in the physical world; you don't get something for nothing. With each stimulation, the body loses some natural force.

For instance, the narcotic known as caffeine found in coffee, tea, and soda will send a surge of energy through the body while in the bloodstream, however, when the buzz is over, the body's available energy falls proportionately as low as it was high. The price you pay for this high is an extremely disrupted digestive system, an acid condition in the stomach, and with continued use, a need for or addiction to the drug caffeine. Caffeine is a direct cause of lumps and tumors in womens breasts. Drinking alcohol is a seemingly wonderful way to forget all your problems and relax your body. The problem is that when you wake up the next day, your difficulties are still staring you in the face, and your body is worse off than when you first decided upon your "solution." Drinking alcohol is as dumb and wasteful a habit as smoking cigarettes. Alcohol abuse and addiction has destroyed millions of lives and millions of families. Be intelligent, and AVOID ALCOHOL.

If you are suffering from a severe headache or from some other type of malady and what you desire is instant relief, as a rule, you would be much better off taking an herb than a drug. There's nothing wrong with trying to gain a little relief, but do not fool yourself into thinking that relief has anything to do with being healthy. Please do yourself a favor and do not rely on any type of herb or supplement for your well-being.

Is the sun bad for you?

Claiming that the "sun causes cancer" is the same as saying that "water causes drowning." Without the sun there would simply be no life on this planet. The places on the globe where the sun shines the most are the very places where the most rich and profound vegetation and life exists. The closer to the equator one travels, the more abundant the greenery. Not much grows in the polar-regions, and there are only a select few species that exist in these sun-deprived locations. Most plants and vegetation simply cannot survive without the sun. The sun is necessary for our health. Those that avoid the sun entirely are asking for trouble.

There are certain natural, biological necessities for life such as air, water, food, and sunshine. What would you tell someone who told you to "stay away from the air?"

Certainly, the sun can damage your skin if you repeatedly overexpose yourself and allow yourself to be burned. Sticking your head in a pail of water for a couple of minutes could be damaging to your health as well, for that matter. The blanket statements made by our health officials to "stay out of the sun" are a good indication of the insanity that runs rampant in the "health" field.

If you have extremely light skin, you obviously must take some extra caution. It would make sense for you to only go in the sun early or late in the day when the suns rays are less potent. Pay attention to how your skin feels and if you experience a burning sensation, get into some shade or cover yourself up. Your body will tell you when you have had enough sun, all you have to do is pay attention.

Eating according to the Laws of Nature will also provide your skin with a tremendous advantage that cannot be acquired from any lotion or sunblock. I noticed a dramatic difference in the quality and resilience of my skin once I began to abide by the Laws of Nature. You will too.

It is a good idea to get as much of your skin exposed to the sun as possible, especially if your lifestyle does not allow for much time in the outdoors. Most people in civilized society are constantly clothed and indoors for weeks, months, and sometimes years at a time. This is an extremely unhealthy way to live. If you work in an office, make it a point to get yourself outside and expose your skin to the sun as often as you can. Even if you live in a cold climate, you must make the effort to sun yourself on a regular basis, if only for five or ten minutes at a time.

Even during the coldest months of the year, there are days when the sun is shining and the wind is still, and I'm able to get some exposure to the sun without getting cold at all. I often find myself in the park exercising in the dead of winter, with below freezing temperatures, stripping off layer after layer until I am shirt-less and sometimes down to my shorts. I actually find I am not only comfortable, but I actually break a sweat while the sun shines on my skin. This is incredibly invigorating, and I find I feel quite revitalized and spirited after these sessions. Be wary of overexposure to frigid temperatures as such exposure is enervating and can cause illness. (With some disciplined training of the mind you can get used to some very cold temperatures and always stay well.)

Nude sunbathing is recommended, but unfortunately, our society frowns upon such a practice. Nonetheless, it is a very good idea to allow the sun to shine on your entire body even if only for a few minutes.

Stay away from all sun-blocks and chemical products as they are pointless and dangerous. When you are in the sun, your skin pores open up and take in these chemical agents and toxins If you're concerned about sun damage to your skin, simply be reasonable and limit your exposure.

Should I drink a lot of water?

There is a common belief that drinking 6 to 8 glasses of water a day is a healthy practice and that "flushing out" the body is beneficial. This a myth created by misunderstanding. First of all, why does your body need to be flushed out? . . . and second of all, just what is it you are flushing?

Hydropathy, or the "water cure," was utilized by the original hygienists. Dr. Sylvester Graham, Dr. Russell Trall, Dr. Isaac Jennings, and Dr. George Field all utilized this technique healing their sick patients. The program originated in nature and practiced by all sick and injured animals, consists of taking no food plus drinking water to satisfy any thirst and keep the eliminative organs running. This is called FASTING and is THE most effective way to return a body to health. When taking no food, we should drink small amounts of water. Because of cessation of eating and the absence of water obtained through fruits and vegetables, our bodies are in need of water.

The point that needs to be clarified is that it is not the water that makes a body well but the cessation of food and the purging of poisons that inevitably takes place when the digestive system is resting. To reiterate, when the digestive system is at rest, the eliminative organs utilize the unused nerve energy to clean the body. The water taken during a fast is simply a way to allow the body to operate without ingesting and digesting food. The water is not healing, curing, or flushing; it is simply aiding the body in its efforts to restore order and well being.

Of course, these doctors and patients experienced tremendous success in allowing the body to heal itself as the body is quite good at it, but for the past hundred years or more the misunderstanding that water is a curative agent has grown to become another "reality" that has little to do with the truth. The idea that drinking massive amounts of water will improve your health is absurd.

Drinking large amounts of water is not a healthy practice, and puts undue strain on the kidneys, and can cause kidney stones. It is also important not to drink water while eating as the water can negate enzyme activity and disturb the digestive process. If you are eating mostly raw foods, you will never have to concern yourself about water intake as most fruits and vegetables are made up of mostly water.

One of the most horrendous crimes against the unknowing public is the lethal array of toxins commonly dumped into our water supplies. Chlorine was one of the first chemical weapons ever used in war (World War I) to burn out the guts of the enemy. It is a highly toxic anti-biological substance put in the water ostensibly for our protection against bacteria.

"We are quite convinced, that there is an association between cancer and chlorinated water."

—Medical College of Wisconsin research team

Fluoride, an aluminum byproduct, is the number one ingredient in rat poison. If you have any doubt about the toxicity of fluoride, you can take a look at the large container of fluoride your dentist has in his office and you will see quite clearly the international sign for poison, the skull and crossbones. Not only does fluoride not keep your teeth strong, it will destroy them and your bones. According to Dr. Dean Burke at the National Cancer

Institute, over 60,000 people each year succumb to cancer caused by ingesting this crippling toxin. Read Dr. John Yiamouyiannis' book *Fluoride the Aging Factor* to find out more about the treachery of this industrial waste pawned off as a health elixir.

The cleanest water on the planet is steam distilled water. Avoid chemically distilled water and be wary of mineral water, as some contain inorganic compounds. For washing your fruits and vegetables, it would make great sense to buy a high-quality water purifier. There are many on the market that can take at least 90% of the chlorine out as well as remove a large amount of heavy metals.

Some states, allow as much as 49% of tap water to be mixed in with the bottled water, without having to inform the buyer. Tap water is filled with many other toxins and industrial wastes other than fluoride and chlorine, including lead and many inorganic compounds. If you are serious about your health, you will avoid tap water at all costs.

Avoid drinking water out of plastic bottles. Many studies have found thousands of chemicals in the water that mimics the effects of potent pharmaceuticals found in numerous brands of commercially sold plastic bottles.

Endocrine Disrupting Chemicals (EDC's) are man made chemicals that interfere with human hormones in both men and women and cause serious health problems such as stunted growth, early puberty, premature birth, infertility and early menopause. These EDC's are found in most plastic bottled water.

(Read the study done by the Plos One medical journal, Aug 28th 2013)

Your best bet is to get a glass water bottle and fill it up with filtered water or bottled steam-distilled water.

CHAPTER

8

NEAT THINGS TO EAT

What do you eat?

This really doesn't matter. What I eat has no bearing on what the Laws of Nature proclaim. If I ate steak with chocolate sauce and chased it with bourbon for every meal, it would not take away from the truth of how human beings were meant to nourish themselves, or from the truth of the knowledge you find in this book. If I decide one day that I want to include cooked foods in my regime, it would not change the natural facts. The point is that personal habits and preferences do not affect what is law. I preface this section with these statements because I have seen and continue to see and hear people who claim to have some *special insight* and create their own personalized *versions* of Nature's Laws to either suit their taste-buds and lifestyles or their pocketbooks.

Nonetheless, I understand the genuine interest of those who are looking to make this transition, so here it is.

I eat nothing but sun-cooked, raw food, except for maybe a few times a year when I will have some cooked vegan food. A normal day of eating might look like this:

Breakfast

I do not eat breakfast or take ANY food before noon.

Lunch

My first meal of the day (around 1 or 2 PM) and usually consists of the tastiest juicy fruits available, such as (in order of preference): bananas, avocados, mangoes, oranges, pears, and/or grapefruit. I'll try to eat only one type of these fruits and may eat two to four of them, depending on how hungry I may be. If I am not quite satiated I may add a couple of extra bananas and/or avocados.

Snacks

Bananas, avocados, oranges, apples, raw unsalted nuts or seeds. Most common for me to snack on are sunflower seeds, pistachios, macadamia nuts, pecans or cashews. Always raw, always unsalted.

Dinner

The biggest meal of my day, my dinner consists of a large salad. The ingredients are:

Avocado (2 or 3), Tomatoes (2 or 3), Cucumber (1), Sprouts (alfalfa, onion, etc.), a red or yellow Pepper, and dulse seaweed . . . absolutely delicious.

Some additional options on this salad include pears, apples, zucchini, spinach, dulse leafs, sunflower seeds, raisins, chives, lemon juice, orange juice, grapefruit, or a mixture. Try throwing a mango in the blender with orange and lemon juice for an exquisite dressing!

Avoid vinegar as it is a ferment, contains acetic acid and will completely disrupt the digestion process and cause other foods in the stomach to turn bad.

Once a week I take a day off from eating for at least 24 hours. Eating so simply affords me a lot of extra time throughout my day. Unlike most people of our culture, I am not bound by meal times or the enslaving urge to not miss a meal. The idea that human beings need to eat three meals a day plus snacks is just not true. This over-feeding is a form of comfort, is an addiction, and is in fact, a major cause of dis-ease.

Eating according to the Laws of Nature and not the laws of culture, or your addictions will create a significant amount of freedom in many areas of your life, as any simpli-fying efforts usually do. Eating in this manner you will begin to catch a glimpse of the wasted time spent thinking about, planning for, preparing, and cleaning up after our meals as well as all the time spent recovering from them in sickness.

What a tremendous gift to find a simpler way to live that will provide some space in your life. Here are some suggestions for those who are interested in making these new food choices and might want a few examples of what it looks like to eat raw food. If you plan to make the change, it is vital that you keep your kitchen counter stocked with your favorite fresh produce. I also suggest getting rid of all your "non-foods" to make room for the new.

Remember to buy organic and to make sure your fruit is always ripe and not too ripe. As a rule, it is NOT a good idea to refrigerate your fruit unless it is in danger of becoming overripe. In a short time, you will become an expert at picking fruits and vegetables. You can also view my YouTube videos "Health Tips With Matthew Grace" on how to pick out fruits and vegetables. For now, it is a good idea to seek out your local green grocer to ask for tips on picking the best produce. Remember there over three hundred varieties of different fruits! Be adventurous and try some things your old self would usually avoid.

As far as equipment goes, you may want to invest in an electric citrus juicer, that will make orange, grapefruit, and lemon juice very quickly. I have used the one made by the Braun company, and I am very happy with it as it is relatively cheap, works great, and takes just a few minutes to clean. Of course, you could just use a regular hand juicer if you want to keep your equipment really simple. If you expect the transition to the natural diet to be difficult, or if you just want to increase your food choices, you may want to invest in a vegetable juicer. There are so many on the market now so it is hard to say which one is best. I will say that for the past 20 years or so I have not heard one complaint from the many people who have been using the Champion juicer. This juicer can make every vegetable juice AND turn any nut into freshly made nut butter, which is quite delicious. This juicer is extremely durable and will last forever. Make sure you have a blender, and you may want to invest in a food processor.

Breakfast

It is NOT the most important meal of the day. My suggestion is to keep it light and simple or just skip it altogether. You can get very used to not eating until noon after just a few days of self-discipline. You should avoid eating any condensed foods such as dried fruit, seeds, or nuts and try not to mix anything.

Fresh Orange Juice, Fresh Grapefruit, Fresh Apple Juice.

- Bananas
- Strawberries
- Mango
- Blueberries
- Peaches
- Nectarines
- Pears
- Cantaloupe
- Pineapple
- Watermelon

Lunch

Quick Stuff

- Avocado ◆ Bananas ◆ Oranges
- Honeydew melon ◆ Grapes ◆ Cashews
- Sunflower seeds & Raisins ◆ dried fruit, seeds, and nuts
- Macadamia nuts ◆ design your own trail mix
- Carrot juice mixed with apples and/or celery, spinach, and/or beets
- Melon (you pick) and a banana in a blender— delicious smoothie
- Almond milk: put a handful of blanched almonds in a blender with 10 to 12 ounces of water. Try mixing in a banana or a pear!

Not so quick

Mango salad: Mesculin greens, sliced mango, raisins, carrots, and sunflower seeds. Add lemon, orange, or grapefruit juice for dressing.

Gazpacho soup: In a blender put tomatoes, cucumber, lemon juice, fresh corn, basil, and scallions (optional). Mix. Do not over-blend as this will destroy the chunky texture. Try refrigerating for added refreshment.

If you are in an office job and do not have a lot of time for your meals, it is no problem since eating raw is the easiest way to go. There is nothing quicker or more convenient than an apple, orange, banana, bag of nuts, or raisins. A cantaloupe or a honeydew melon is an entire meal that comes with its own built-in bowl. It is helpful to carry around a good sized pocket knife with a stainless steel blade to cut your fruit.

If you have a business lunch, you can call ahead to make sure they can prepare a salad for you. It is always a good idea to eat before you show up so that you are less tempted to eat something you did not plan to eat.

Dinner

Casaba melon or any other melon with lime juice.

Guacamole: Chopped avocados, tomatoes, lemon and/ or lime juice, and chives. Chop up some cucumber, carrots, zucchini, and celery for dipping.

Matt's Salad: A handful of dulse (seaweed) leaves marinated for 5 minutes underneath 3 chopped tomatoes, 2 chopped avocado, 1 chopped cucumber (I prefer Kirbys'), a garden blend of sprouts (alfalfa, onion, clover, etc.), and some dulse flakes sprinkled on top. I also enjoy some raw corn in this concoction occasionally.

Tomato sauce: Soak a handful of large, pitted dates (about 12) and a large handful of dried tomatoes in purified water for 2 to 3 hrs. Place in a blender or food processor with 3 or 4 chopped, ripe tomatoes and a chopped stalk of celery. Blend until thoroughly mixed. You can cut open avocados and place a dollop of this tomato sauce on either half. Really delicious!

Cuke Salad: Diced cucumbers and tomatoes with dill and lemon juice.

Fruit Salad: Diced mangos, bananas, raisins, and coconut flakes.

Dessert

Ice Cream: If you want a great dessert, try freezing peeled ripe bananas, and putting them in a food processor. You can add a little raw almond butter or tahini (raw ground sesame seeds) as well as some strawberries or blueberries.

Apple pie: *Crust:* Soak a large handful (12 to 15) of pitted dates in purified water for 2 to 3 hours. Drain and put the soaked dates in the food processor. Add about 8 ounces of walnuts and/or pecans and about 8 ounces of sunflower seeds. Mix until they become a thick paste. This is your pie crust that you will spread evenly into your pie dish. It is fine if there are small chunks of nuts and seeds in the crust but make sure the dates are well blended throughout.

Filling: Use your favorite apples (about 4 to 6 fresh apples depending on the size of the apples and the size of your pie dish) mixed evenly with dried apples (about 2 large handfuls), half fresh and half dried. Let your food processor grind them up nicely. Fill your pie crust with the end product, and you have a delicious AND nutritious dessert! You can use thinly sliced apples to garnish your pie. I suggest refrigerating for at least 10 to 15 minutes before serving to help the ingredients bind together.

You can also try different fillings like sliced bananas and/or mangos instead of apples for a raw tropical pie.

This is a very short list of the possibilities that exist for you. I encourage you to experiment for yourself and get creative.

The key to making Raw food recipes is to make them delicious while avoiding using salt in your preparations as ALL salt is toxic and no good for you.

9

MIND, EMOTIONS
AND HEALING

For more than twenty-five years I have been assisting people in their struggle to overcome dis-ease
and achieve health. It has been my experience that the
cessation of poisoning the body and living according
to natural laws is the most effective, and safest way to
restore one's health. By proper feeding and detoxification,
an improvement in one's health is a sure thing. Exercise is
also a requisite and an undisputed aid to health and vigor.
Fresh air, sunshine and the cessation of ALL poisoning
acts will surely lead to a healthier body.

Having a Healthy body will do wonders for your
attitude, emotional well being and disposition. Being
healthy and existing in a pain-free, energized vital body
is an exciting uplifting experience, especially if you have
been sick most of your life. In addition to changing your
diet from the SAD (Standard American Diet), there is

also the opportunity to change the way you think and feel.

How much one improves is directly related to the attitude of the individual. Their "inner stance" and approach towards their physical condition and their extant possibilities have a major effect on the results they achieve. What one believes and tells themselves about the process they are undergoing can either limit the healing or advance them to a full recovery.

We all have witnessed how some people will become so identified with their disease that it becomes the center of their world. Most of their thoughts and conversations revolve around their illness. They use their illness as a means of avoiding life and shirking responsibility, as well as a means of gaining additional attention and sympathy. They are unwilling to hear that recovery is an option and actually will lash out at those that suggest it. There are some people who simply love their disease and wouldn't give it up for anything.

Obviously, if you are reading this book, you are probably sincere about finding a way out of your present condition. (At the same time, it could only help to do a thorough investigation to see if there is some unspoken or unrecognized part of you that enjoys whatever benefit you may get from your illness.) People who love or have a tacit fondness for their disease are unlikely to get well.

For some of you, things may seem hopeless and you may feel defeated. If you feel hopeless, you must fight to have hope. If you feel defeated you must realize that the game is never over until you decide. You must come up in yourself and force yourself to think in affirmative and empowering ways. Most have the response "but what if I fail?" Listen and listen closely. The results of your efforts do not matter. If you never get any better but continue on fighting you are a massive success. Accepting your condition without a fight is the only thing that may be considered a failure. Failure to meet the challenge you have attracted in your life. So all you have to do is get interested in living a rich full life with NO CONCERN FOR THE FUTURE.

You will get some great help here in this chapter. It has been said that we are never given a challenge that is too much for us to handle. View your illness as a test. Accept it. Take it on as a challenge that you must overcome. You can even make a game of it.

THE most important aspect of dealing with disease is THE WISH to overcome it. Hope for a better future.

We have seen those with serious illnesses and physical handicaps who have an unstoppable and heroic spirit. They are all around us. No severity of illness or handicap can prevent them from living their lives. Their disease or handicap IS NOT the center of their attention. They focus on the things they can do and continue to live their lives with an upbeat and positive attitude. What is possible for you is limited only by the way you think and feel.

There are endless inspirational stories of men and women who have overcome great physical challenges: I have seen men with no arms play the guitar, well. You may be thinking "what are you talking about, if they have no arms they can't even hold a guitar." That is true. They play with their feet. Their names are Tony Melendez and Mark Goffeney. Their music is simply wonderful and their technique and sound is amazing. Mr Melendez (a victim of thalidomide, the drug responsible for thousands of severe birth defects) has played for the Pope and was hailed as "An example of Hope for humanity." Goffeney started a band called Big Toe and was signed to a record contract.

There is another young lady born with severe birth defects, she plays the piano like a virtuoso; her name is He Ah Lee, she has no legs and only two fingers on each hand. She does the impossible. I have seen men with no legs run, with prosthetics, as well as any other man. Just check out the Paralympic Games if you ever need any inspiration. Helen Keller, despite not being able to hear or see, lived a rich full life and changed the world for millions of people. I could go on and on with stories of the sick and impaired who overcame their obstacles to have a real Life. You can as well.

Miracles are born of change of perception.

None of the above-mentioned people focused on what they could not do. They shifted their minds and hearts to focus on their possibilities and insisted that their lives would be meaningful and productive. You can do the same. It may take some serious re-wiring of your belief systems and ways of thinking and feeling. You must believe you can do it.

YOU can enjoy proving your doctor wrong. Believe me, it's a lot of fun.

The above is a quote from Dr. Bernie Siegal author of *Love, Medicine and Miracles* and many other wonderful books and articles. Dr. Siegal, who prefers to be called Bernie, attended Colgate University and Cornell University Medical College. He holds membership in two scholastic honor societies, Phi Beta Kappa and Alpha Omega Alpha, and graduated with honors. His surgical training took place at Yale New Haven Hospital and the Children's Hospital of Pittsburgh. He was a pediatric and general surgeon in New Haven.

He has been one of the strongest advocates for patients who have been told that they have no hope. He has helped scores of these people left for dead by the medical world, re-gain their health and live with a completely different approach. He understands that the way we think and feel has a direct, intense and immediate effect on our well-being. He implores his patients to be active in their approach to their illness. He is convinced that a responsible physician will no longer ignore the patient's emotional and intellectual life. He believes that a doctor who is genuinely interested in the well being of his patient must get to know that person's emotional and intellectual makeup. I highly recommend his books.

> *"I see people who die a few minutes after a doctor tells them there is no hope of a cure. They give up and go. Others get angry and find joy in proving the doctor wrong. Something within them is challenged and hopeful. Hope is the divine motivator."*
>
> — DR. BERNIE SIEGAL

Hope is the most important factor in our lives and this is demonstrated by the common occurrence of an elderly spouse dying within a few days of their loved one's death, often times with no serious or life-threatening affliction of their own. All hope for the future is gone and the life force is extinguished in the surviving spouse.

If you have ANY doubt that your beliefs systems, thought patterns and emotions are vital to your recovery and/or your well being all you have to do is look at the research done on the placebo effect. All doubts will go out the window.

Placebo effect

Placebo (Latin for I will please) trials are commonly used in the "double blind" form where neither patient nor doctor knows if the drug being dispensed to a group of patients is inert or the actual drug being tested. Over the years it has been proved that at least 30% of the time the inert, or fake pill works to alleviate or end the symptoms.

Obviously, the patients' thoughts and feelings about the inert bread or sugar pill given to them by the physician is what activates the body's healing powers. What other explanation could there be?

Dr. Herbert Benson from Harvard University believes that placebos work up to 90% of the time. Whether it is 30% or 90% or somewhere in between it is none the less a remarkable phenomenon that we really need to pay more attention to.

In the book, *The Psychobiology of Mind-Body Healing*, written by Ernest Lawrence Rossi, we find the following mention about the 55–60% placebo connection, "In other words, the effectiveness of placebo compared to standard doses of different analgesic drugs under double-blind circumstances seems to be relatively constant . . . it is worth noting that this 56% effectiveness ratio is not limited to placebo versus analgesic drugs. It is also found in double-blind studies of non-pharmacological insomnia treatment techniques (58% from 14 studies) and psychotropic drugs for the treatment of depression such as tricyclics (59% from 93 studies reviewed by Morris & Beck, 1974) and lithium (62% from 13 studies reviewed in Marini, Sheard, Bridges and Wagner, 1976). Thus, it appears that placebo is about 55–60% as effective as active medications irrespective of the potency of these active medications."

"In a study of morphine, there was a 50% pain reduction in 75% of the patients treated. The placebo group had a 50% pain reduction in 36% of the patients."

In 1980 there were over 1000 articles dealing with placebos. Placebos had a high rate of activity in the areas of coughing, mood swings, diabetes, anxiety, asthma, sarcoma, dermatitis, headaches, rheumatoid arthritis, radiation sickness, Multiple Sclerosis and Parkinson's.

A group of patients was told they were given LSD when in fact they were given the placebo. They had all the physiological effects noted with LSD.

Dr. David Sobel, a placebo specialist with Kaiser hospital told the following: "a doctor was treating one of his asthma patients with a new drug. This new potent medicine worked within minutes. When the patient had the next attack the doctor gave the placebo. The man complained it didn't work. Then the doctor received a letter that stated the first pill was actually a placebo that was sent by mistake." More from Ernest Lawrence:

"Ipecac is a substance known to always induce vomiting. A 28-year-old female who was suffering from two straight days of nausea and vomiting was given 10cc of Ipecac syrup and told it was a new drug that stopped vomiting. In twenty minutes the vomiting had stopped completely. Her stomach showed normal contractive activity."

"During a study for headaches, 120 of our 199 patients receiving the placebo obtained relief. In a test of Clofibrate versus placebo for cholesterol level and cardiovascular mortality, the placebo outperformed the drug."

"Placebos effectiveness is in proportion to what the doctor and the patient think they are using. Two placebo pills are better than one and an injection always seems to be more effective than a pill. Placebo capsules are more effective than tablets. When placebos are administered, the yellow and orange are great for mood manipulators, the dark red as a sedative; white as painkillers and lavender as hallucinogens."

"In a back pain sham therapy of four years, 40% of the placebo group improved."

"In a sham tooth-grinding surgical procedure, there was a 64% total symptom remission."

"Doctors Seidel and Abrams found that a hypodermic of saline was as effective as vaccines for chronic rheumatoid arthritis."

"In a study for Raynaud's Syndrome, utilizing an apparatus with saline and the clicking of dials, every case using the placebo improved. Six had excellent improvement and one patient great improvement after one year."

Astonishing. Why aren't more research dollars invested to study of the power of the mind and emotions?

It may have to do with the fact that changing the way you think and feel is free. There are no profits to be made.

The author presents three case histories of patients with multiple personality disorder. One client was found to be allergic to citrus fruits in all personality states save one; the allergic response was abruptly terminated by switching to a different personality. The second client was severely allergic to cats, except in one personality state in which she could play with cats indefinitely with no rash, lacrimation, or wheezing. The third responded to cigarette smoke with marked dyspnea and asthmatic bronchospastic wheezing in one personality and was totally free of symptoms in a smoky environment in a second personality.[1]

Braun BG. Psychophysiologic phenomena in multiple personality and hypnosis. Am J Clin Hypn. 1983; 26(2):124–37.

---

1   From *Bruno Klopfer, Psychological Variables in Human Cancer, Journal of Prospective Techniques 31, 1957, pp. 331–40.*

A study in England was done where 100 men were told that they were taking chemotherapy when in actuality they were taking inactive saline solution, 20% of these men lost their hair.

In an experiment conducted by Dr. Joan Borysenko, co-founder and director of the mind/body clinic, it was found that 30% of women lost their hair when told they were being given chemotherapy, despite the fact they were given a placebo.

How powerful are our thoughts and feelings?

One of the most astounding examples of suggestible healing comes from psychologist Bruno Klopfer who was treating a man who had advanced cancer in his lymph nodes. The patient's name was Mr. Wright and he had tried every conventional treatment available and he was very close to death. His neck, armpits, chest, abdomen, and groin were filled with tumors the size of oranges, and his spleen and liver were so enlarged that two quarts of milky fluid had to be drained out of his chest every day.

> "Wright heard about an exciting new drug called Krebiozen, and he begged his doctor to let him try it. At first, the doctor refused because the drug was being tried on people with a life expectancy of at least three months. Nonetheless, the doctor gave in and gave Wright an injection of the Krebiozen on a Friday, but thought that Mr. Wright would be dead in a couple of days."
>
> "The following Monday he found Wright out of bed and walking around. Klopfer reported that his tumors had 'melted like snowballs on a

hot stove and were half their original size. Ten days after Wright's first treatment, he left the hospital and was, as far as his doctors could tell, cancer free. When he entered the hospital he had needed an oxygen mask to breathe, but when he left, he was well enough to fly his own plane at 12,000 feet with no discomfort."

"Wright remained well for about two months, but then articles began to appear asserting that Krebiozen actually had no effect on cancer of the lymph nodes. Wright, who was rigidly logical and scientific in his thinking, became very depressed, suffered a relapse, and was readmitted to the hospital. This time his physician decided to try an experiment. He told Wright that Krebiozen was every bit as effective as it had seemed, but that some of the initial supplies of the drug had deteriorated during shipping. He explained, however, that he had a new highly concentrated version of the drug and could treat Wright with this. The physician used only plain water and went through an elaborate procedure before injecting Wright with the placebo.

"Again the results were dramatic. Tumor masses melted, chest fluid vanished, and Wright was quickly back on his feet and feeling great. He remained symptom-free for another two months, but then the AMA announced that a nationwide study of Krebiozen had found the drug worthless for the treatment of cancer. This time Wright's faith was completely shattered.

His cancer blossomed anew and he died two days later."

Are there any limits of our healing powers when our mind and emotions join in? Are the beliefs "I am sick and dying" and "there is no hope for me" the actual cause of death? In Mr. Wright's case evidently so. What is possible for us when thinking and feeling in a clear effective manner? Remember the people in these medical trials were not consciously trying to evoke a set of beliefs or think with any intention at all, and they got better. They assumed they were taking effective medicine and it worked.

What about the patients who did not respond to the placebo? Perhaps they had no real belief one way or another or in fact, doubted that the treatment would work. What if these patients were given some training on how to think about their treatment and illness? What if we could, through rigorous mental exercises (visualization, meditation, etc.), begin to gain control over the mind and emotions? What if we were able to train our minds to think with intention, to ignore any and all harmful debilitating thoughts and feelings and to think and feel precisely what is needed for our recovery and nothing else? Instead of being content with our ordinary mental laziness where we "think" whatever arbitrary and useless thought happens to pop into our head and get swept away with any random emotion we presently feel, perhaps it is possible to choose what we think and what we feel. Just as eliminating the physical poisons from our bodies we could eliminate the intellectual and emotional poisons.

Is it possible we could *think* ourselves back to health?

For a little more extreme, yet well-documented evidence of what our incredible human bodies are capable of when in a certain mental/emotional state:

In eighteenth-century Paris, subsequent to the death of Father Francois de Paris, leader of a heretical group of Catholics called Jansenists, his followers began ritualistic gatherings at his grave site. All types of miraculous healing took place.

The Catholic Church and the ruling monarch, Louis XV perceived the Jansenists as a threat to their power. The king sent men to see what was going on and to report back to him how the Jansenists were fooling people into believing in miracles. He was astonished that the investigators confirmed the miracles as fact. The Church then declared that the Jansenists were doing the work of the devil. Then Louis XV tried to close the cemetery where Father de Paris was buried, François-Marie Arouet Voltaire, the famous French Enlightenment author and philosopher who was one of many renowned witnesses to the miracles was reported to say, "God is forbidden by order of the King to perform any more miracles in the cemetery of Saint-Medard."

The miracles continued and often the participants were seized by strange spasms that earned them the name *convulsionnaires*. Certain participants reportedly became clairvoyant while others levitated. Strangest of all, however, while in this convulsive state the Jansenists became completely indestructible, letting the strongest men try to strangle them, spear them, burn them, hammer iron nails through their stomachs, pound their bodies hundreds of times with sledgehammers, and drop heavy stone weights from high overhead directly onto their bodies—all with no signs of physical injury. Often times the men and women would cry out to their torturers "hit me harder." The King then sent a battalion of men to the cemetery to destroy the Jansenists, they failed miserably. The officer who was in command of those men left for England to write about the experience.

These events were witnessed by hundreds of people including David Hume the Scottish philosopher. He went on to write in his Philosophical Essays:

> "*There surely never was so great a number of miracles ascribed to one person as those which were lately said to have been wrought in France upon the tomb of Abbe Paris. Many of the miracles were immediately proven on the spot, before judges of unquestioned credit and distinction, in a learned age, and on the most eminent theatre that is now in the world.*"

Basil Carre de Montgeron, an established member of the French Parliament was witness to so many of these miracles that he began writing about them and documenting these incredible feats. He published four very thick volumes in 1737, La Verite des Miracles, about the feats of the Jansenists. The church continued to view these miracles as a threat to their own power, however, The Catholic Encyclopedia today has this to say about the Jansenist miracles:

"But what was more astonishing was that their bodies, subjected during the crises to all sorts of painful tests, seemed at once insensible and invulnerable; they were not wounded by the sharpest instruments, or bruised by enormous weights or blows of incredible violence . . . Several of the so-called miraculous cures were proved (to be) based only on testimonies which were either false, interested, preconcerted, and more than once retracted, or at least valueless, the echoes of disease and fanatic imaginations . . . On the other hand, although fraud was discovered in several cases, it is impossible to attribute them all indiscriminately to trickery or ignorant simplicity. Critically speaking, the authenticity of some extraordinary phenomena is beyond question, as they took place publicly and in the presence of reliable witnesses."

Obviously, the Jansenists are extreme examples of how certain emotions can alter, transform and protect our bodies. The fact that these people became nearly indestructible in this state leads me to wonder if dis-ease in the body could be completely eradicated if we were able to think and feel in an effective way.

For seven years I competed as heavyweight boxer and thought it very interesting that fighters "got used" to getting hit in the face and the body. I actually had the experience hundreds and hundreds of times of getting hit with clean blows and feeling little or no pain AND not a mark left on the face. Someone in a street fight who gets hit with one punch usually experiences serious pain and will have a big swollen, black and blue eye immediately. In a normal competitive sparring session, a good fighter may get hit with 3 or 4 clean hard blows (that would knock most people out cold) and about 20 to 30 glancing blows that would send a normal person reeling and seriously hurt them. Yet, often times there will not be a mark on this fighter's face. What is that? And why on certain days did I feel acute pain from punches landed and other days almost nothing? It certainly didn't have to do with the opponent I was fighting with or sparring with as I often sparred with the same lot of fighters.

I remember one particular sparring session. I was in the ring with a heavy puncher, who I had many tough and grueling sparring sessions with, who invariably would catch me with big blows, especially his overhand right. He had good power and I always felt it. This four-round session stood out as it had a magical quality to it. Not only could none of his sledge-hammer right hands hurt me but everything was different. Breathing was very easy and effortless throughout the four rounds, a rare occurrence in such a grueling, intense situation. I felt an extreme sense of relaxation. The astounding thing was that time changed. All the speed and furious action that was taking place I was experiencing all in a strange sort of slow motion. Not only could I see every punch coming at me and easily avoid it. I was able to land my combinations with pinpoint accuracy. The few punches he did land felt like nothing. I mean nothing, as if a little girl was hitting me. It was astonishing. It got to the point where I actually had to back off as the sparring session became too one-sided.

Obviously, that was a rare and unique state. Maybe something like the Jansenists experienced. I tried to recreate that experience the rest of my boxing career without much success. In fact, we boxed again the next day and it was as grueling and ordinary as ever. I got hit with about 5–6 hard shots and they all hurt.

That incredible state of physical consciousness I previously experienced was real. I did feel close to indestructible. And I have never forgotten it and other similar experiences.

Another experience of mine stands out regarding mind over matter. I was in the gym lifting weights. Doing seated rows (upper back exercise) with over two hundred pounds. I made an amateurish mistake at the end of the set that caused a severe pain in my lower back. In fact, I not only felt the tear, I HEARD the tear. At the time I had been studying a lot about the mind and its effects on the body. About how powerful the idea of "ACTING AS IF" can be. I had been experimenting with myself and my clients, and had recently done a couple of mind-body tests; a couple of fire-walks with great success (no burns) and stood out in 20 degrees (F) weather for four hours in only a dress shirt without getting sick.

As I released the weight I screamed out, the pain shot from my back and my face and body contorted in agony. Being an athlete my entire life I knew what a significant injury felt like. This was one. My training partner looked with alarm knowing full well I was injured. I thought about how this is going to affect me and my workouts for the coming weeks and I got angry and felt stupid about my poor form. My mind had caught up quickly with my body and within a second or two I remembered what I had been learning about mind power and immediately began to change my state.

I began to breathe as if I was fine, deepening the short shallow breaths of a man in pain. I stood up as if I was fine and was at once stabbed back down by the nerve-endings in the lower left small of the back. I held onto my knees in a bent over position. My face contorted again but I relaxed it immediately. I told my training partner who was very concerned, as calmly and as seriously as I could, to leave me alone and to go ahead and finish his workout without me. I did not want someone acting as if I was hurt while trying to act as if I was fine. My aim was to act as if I was fine AND to complete my back workout.

Upon straightening up, breathing deeply and relaxing as best as I could I had to counter all of the mechanical thoughts that rush in at such a moment "lie down immediately, get in the hot shower, put some ice on it, get some help" and many others. Along with the mental pictures of causing a bit of a scene at the gym, hobbling home, missing workouts, being upset or angry etc.

"I AM FINE." I repeated over and over again as I began to slowly walk around the gym. ACTING AS IF I had just arrived and was really looking forward to my training session. I walked away from the seated row machine where my training partner was watching me from across the gym with a look of confusion. My face must have turned white as a couple of people (who didn't see what happened) asked me if I was alright. "I am fine," I said, happy to affirm out loud without looking like a weirdo.

There was a real fight for my mind between the mechanical thoughts and what I was consciously willing AND what the pain coursing through my body was saying. I had to get rid of the residual effect of fear and alarm that was still palpable in my bloodstream, that sense of fear and dread. By the time I got to the other side of the gym it could have gone either way. Here existed a very strange mental phenomenon. A part of me KNEW what my goal was and the other part did not. It was passive and helpless against the conscious willing part. At the same time, there was a third part of me that saw both parts.

I kept increasing my efforts to relax and to think the thoughts I normally think when entering the gym. I started to speak to someone and noticed after a thirty-second conversation they saw no pain on my face worth mentioning, and I relaxed a little more despite the knife in my back. My voice sounded normal and I said nothing out of the ordinary. Good. I was in great pain and kept moving from one side of the long gym floor to the other and nobody asked again if I was ok. By the second trip across the hard rubber floor, I began to feel an ease of the level 10 pain (1–10 pain scale) down to about an 8 and there was no looking back. It took about 10 to 15 minutes of "Acting As If" before I decided to do a very light exercise for my forearms.

I picked up a 35lb barbell carefully, but also with insistent confidence that I was fine. One part of my brain actively affirming while another recessed part of the brain thinking "am I nuts?" Am I going to pick up this barbell and end on the floor writhing in pain?" And "Am I really this stupid, trying to do this when I know I am hurt?" I brought it over to a vacant bench and put it on the floor, already realizing that something was happening. With my legs on either side of the bench, I bent over and picked up the bar. A sharp but bearable pain was met with a deep breath and increased affirmations as I placed my forearms on the bench and began doing wrist curls. "Fourteen, fifteen" and I let the weight drop to the floor. This seemed like a great exercise for the situation as it didn't put direct pressure on the lower back but did, in fact, seem to stretch it out.

After three sets of 15 to 20 reps of wrist curls, the pain was down to a 4 or a 5. My aim was to finish my back workout and all of a sudden it seemed possible! Calm and intense focus was what was needed now. No time to celebrate. I went over to the "t-bar" machine that has a pad where you place your chest and grab a bar at shoulder-width and do a rowing movement. I put on a very lightweight and did one set. Pain level 4. Put a little more weight on (for a total of half of the weight I usually did on that machine) and did three more sets. Confidence was now building alongside the unspoken thought "is this really happening?"

I was really astonished and didn't quite know what to think or say. I said nothing but continued on with my workout, moving in a relaxed manner. I found myself on the seated row machine where the injury occurred about a twenty minutes ago. I put on a very lightweight and did a set with NO PAIN. This was the very machine and the exact same movement that caused the painful, audible tear. I was now moving fine with NO noticeable discomfort or caution in my movements. Internally I was beginning to celebrate, a pretty affirmative state that was only helping. I did three more sets with just a little more weight increasing the number of repetitions and actually feeling that I was exhausting the targeted muscles. I realized that although I halved the amount of weight used, I had technically finished my back workout.

I was ecstatic and amazed and wondered if I was lying to myself about how bad I was hurt, or if I was maybe in some state of shock and was about to go to the hospital. I was afraid to talk about it for a few reasons. The first being that talking about an injury is part of the mechanical reaction and I wanted to continue on doing the opposite.

I walked home with no physical discomfort and did my best to continue to affirm while a faint voice continued to wonder if all hell was going to break loose. I slept great that night with only the slightest of twinges in my back. The next morning there was no pain! Just an ever slight tightness as a reminder of the injury that healed immediately. I met my training partner the next day for our shoulder workout and he said: "Man, I thought you were going to the hospital after that set."

Looking back on this experience I am convinced that if I went with my normal mental, physical and emotional reactions I would have experienced days, if not weeks of pain and debilitation. I know this is anecdotal evidence of mind over matter but it was a genuine experience that helped me to shape how I think and feel. This experience helped form the way I think about my possibilities. This event bolstered my belief in the fact that we have tremendous possibilities and control over our bodies, far more than we imagine.

Last year I dropped a 90 lb dumbbell on my toe. It was agonizingly painful (and quite embarrassing). I did everything I wrote about above and finished my workout and recovered without ever seeing a doctor or getting it X rayed. It DID hurt a lot but I fully recovered in a couple of days and did not miss any work.

One night I was scheduled to compete in the NYC Golden Gloves while having a fever of 103 degrees and feeling very sick. I had seriously over trained and was quite broken down. It was brutal trying to get emotionally and physically prepared to fight. Getting to the arena I felt like an idiot as I felt like collapsing while on the subway. Getting up the stairs to the street felt like a marathon. I was burning up as I got dressed and had my hands taped. Once the bell sounded I was fine. As soon as the fight was over I felt horrible and stayed in bed for two days. Obviously, I had the same body during the fight than I did before and afterward. I did not feel sick during the fight. I also had to fight a 3 round fight one night with a broken jaw. I won each of these fights and was able to perform very well despite the illness and injury. The mind is a powerful tool.

Additionally, it is clear and everyone can have their own evidence, that if we begin to utilize our mind and apply intentional thought with consistency and intensity we CAN change our bodies, affect our health and decrease if not completely eliminate pain.

In fact, people who have multiple personalities have completely different responses to allergens when changing from one personality to the next. In one personality they are extremely allergic and their bodies have acute responses breaking out in hives, and having difficulty breathing. They switch to another personality and their symptoms vanish. This is an astonishing occurrence that has been well documented in many different cases through the years. These people obviously have the same bodies yet completely different results when in different personalities. This is confirmation that the way we think and feel directly changes our body's chemistry. Also, that our thoughts and emotions are the most important aspects in creating dis-ease or health. What is personality other than a long list of acquired beliefs, thoughts, emotions, physical posture, and habits? If someone with multiple personalities can completely eradicate their symptoms by "changing personalities" it is my strong contention that we can do the same.

What if a person who is very sick decided to drop ALL beliefs about themselves along with all their habitual "thinking" and feeling? Think of your thoughts, feelings, postures and ways of being as "ingredients" for a recipe for disease. Well if there is a recipe for disease there MUST be a recipe for Health. What if you began to observe the way you breathe, hold yourself, speak to others, speak to yourself, your inner dialogue, the type of words you chose etc. Chances are you will find that you are actually partaking in the creation of dis-ease in the body. It is imperative NOT to judge yourself but to simply OBSERVE these habits without the reactionary mind.

After a while of simple observation, you can begin to alter your state by changing the way you breathe, walk, sit and move in general. You can begin to change the thoughts you think and begin to think with intention. You can become a guardian to yourself and refuse to allow ANY negative thoughts or emotions to take hold of you be it envy, hatred, jealousy, shame, depression, fear etc. If you feel depression setting in STOP what you are doing. Look Up. (It is physiologically impossible to be depressed while looking up.) Start exercising or go for a brisk walk.

Breathe Deeply. Depression requires shallow breathing. Put on some inspiring music. Dance. REFUSE to go with the negativity. This takes a lot of effort and a lot of practice but is incredibly rewarding. Eventually, you will become a different person. You will be adding new ingredients and be rewarded with a completely different result.

Louise Hay author of *You Can Heal your Life* offers keen insight into how our diseases and physical afflictions are caused by our emotions. For every affliction, she offers affirmations to practice and say aloud and to yourself. This is the beginning of mentally and emotionally re-wiring ourselves for health. Her books are very helpful to anyone looking to overcome disease. I recommend her book *You Can Heal Your Life*.

We have been given the short sell on our possibilities as human beings. We have been kept in the dark about our potential and what we can achieve. We really need to begin to understand just what is possible for us, no matter what our doctor says, or what the common beliefs of the day happen to be.

Dr. Robert Ornstein from the University of California, claims that the number of possible connections in the brain (neuron to neuron) is greater than the number of atoms in the universe!

Psychologically speaking, we could use the analogy that we are living in a small three foot by three-foot dark corner in the dungeon of a 50,000 square foot mansion. We think our dark corner is our entire house and seem to be comfortable and satisfied as most people are living in similar dark corners. It is obvious to me that we were meant to live in the palace.

Some cancer patients receiving the ultra-toxic and deadly "chemotherapy" and radical surgeries actually survive despite the toxic barrage on their body and go on to live normal lives. Most people die from the "treatment."

> "I have seen patients who have been paralyzed by cobalt spine radiation, and after vitamin treatment, their HCG test is faintly positive. We got their cancer, but the radiogenic manipulation is such that they can't walk . . . It's the cobalt that will kill, not the cancer."
> —Letter from John Richardson, M.D., to G. Edward Griffin, dated Dec. 2, 1972; Griffin, Private Papers, op. cit.)

Radiation "therapy" has the extra distinction of also spreading the very cancer it is supposed to combat. If the patient does survive the radiation then his body still faces a monstrous battle. Once the cancer has metastasized to a second location, their chance of survival is greatly diminished.

The point is, I contend that the ones who survive cancer and cancer treatments have an intense belief that they are going to recover and they get better in spite of the "treatments," I do not think for one second that ANY form of health is achieved by these highly toxic, bio-destructive "treatments" or radical surgeries. I do however suppose that if one were to completely believe in the treatments and their doctors that their chances of survival are greatly increased. A positive attitude towards one's recovery makes all the difference.

Emotions

Just as in the physical realm, where it is not so much the addition of anything new that restores one's health but the subtraction of harmful practices that restores health, it may be the same emotionally. To begin with, it may be wise if we state what emotions are harmful to our physical apparatus: Envy, hate, resentment, worry, grandiosity, selfishness, jealousy, and anger literally eat our health away. Anyone who has made the effort to begin to observe the effects of these invisible poisons will testify to their pernicious effects on the body.

Resentment is like taking poison and hoping someone else dies. Repressed, unaddressed anger leads to depression. Envy and jealousy make you feel less than. Stop comparing yourself to others. Worry is a useless emotion that does ONLY harm to the one who worries and all who come in contact with you. Worry has only to do with what has happened or what will happen. Although many of us think it is a way to "show how much we care." Worry is not a sufficient substitute for love. Stop it if you wish to be healthy. Living in the moment is the cure for worry and guarantees increased health. Considering others and helping others is also a cure for these mental venoms. All of these emotions are actually disease producers.

Most doctors and scientists do not consider the emotions or thoughts of their patients as being a factor in the cause, prevention or eradication of disease. Understandably, as it is not yet possible to weigh a thought or an emotion or measure their size or shape. You cannot take an emotion or a thought, put it on a petri dish and examine it under a microscope. Most doctors will not ask their patients questions like "how is your life going?" or "can you tell me what's on your mind?" Your doctor will stick to the physical realm only. Unfortunately he/she is limited in the treatment offered, drugs or surgery. Both of these options treat only the symptoms of disease, not the cause. Both create more problems than you originally had.

Also, teaching people how to think and feel in different ways to create health is really not good for business.

Most doctors are completely unprepared to make an emotional connection with their patients. It is obviously not an important part of their training in medical school and is certainly not a priority in the hospital environment. I cannot tell you the depths of awkwardness, ignorance, and irresponsibility I have seen from doctors when dealing with their patients. One doctor, in particular, telling a patient, who was a friend of mine "you are getting worse." That man died a week later. I have witnessed certain doctors speak to their patients with boundless recklessness and think nothing of it. I have experienced first hand the baneful bedside manners of physicians wondering if they ever heard the Hippocratic Oath they took: First Do No Harm.

I have also noticed that the most successful and revered doctors are those who know how to connect emotionally with the people they are treating. They create a genuine connection that makes the patient feel relaxed and confident.

There are a few highly qualified doctors who are stating very clearly that thoughts and emotions play more than an incidental role in the creation of health or disease.

The great back doctor, Dr. John Sarno from New York writes in his book, *Healing Back Pain: The Mind Body Connection:*

> "It has been my observation that the majority of these pain syndromes are the result of a condition in the muscles, nerves tendons and ligaments brought on by tension."

Dr. Sarno has helped thousands of people recover from severe and crippling back pain despite X-ray and MRI evidence of structural damage, by revealing to his patients that their minds and emotions are the cause of their physical pain. He calls it Tension Myositis. I highly recommend his books.

I am convinced, as are thousands of others, that what Dr. Sarno says is absolutely correct. I also believe that the mind-body(emotion) connection can be taken much further than back pain, into every other aspect of disease and recovery.

It seems impossible to achieve good health while having a center of gravity in negativity. At the same time, the counter seems to be true: A person with a loving, forgiving and generous heart seems always to be thriving physically. Even when injured or sick, they retain a sense of humor and/or a fighting spirit. In fact, it is rare to find an individual who is in love and not feeling well. I have interviewed scores of people who cannot remember ever being sick while in the throes of love. Of course, that wonderful, dreamlike state of being in love may be a great way to ensure health but how does one live in such a high state with any kind of consistency? It may be possible but it is not likely that that particular degree of intensity can last. However, there are degrees of positive emotions that are attainable and sustainable. One is simply being more optimistic.

Here is some scientific evidence that the way we view ourselves and our world affects our health. It may be worth it to take on a more optimistic approach to our lives. A study done in May 2008 by the Harvard Men's Health Watch is quite interesting.

According to a series of studies, optimists enjoy better health than pessimists. The May 2008 issue of *Harvard Men's Health Watch* explores possible reasons for this connection.

Many studies have reported that optimism influences health. Among the findings:

- Optimistic coronary bypass patients were only half as likely as pessimists to require re-hospitalization.
- Highly pessimistic men were three times more likely to develop hypertension.
- People with positive emotions had lower blood pressures.

In one study, the most pessimistic men were more than twice as likely to develop heart disease compared with the most optimistic.

Anyone who suffers from ulcers knows quite clearly that being tense or angry exacerbates this condition. "Flare ups" coincide with their emotional state. We actually have a name used for a certain kind of headache known as a "tension headache." The tension caused by our thinking and feeling a certain way. Soldiers who have been in battle are often diagnosed with "post-traumatic stress disorder." Despite the fact there is no physical examination that will reveal this condition, modern medicine recognizes this as a legitimate medical condition (once known as "shell shocked").

Carolyn Myss (pronounced Mase) a medical intuitive, has been writing and teaching about the effects of our emotions on our health. Her work was a big help to me in my physical recovery. She has been working with Harvard-trained neurosurgeon and researcher Dr. Norman Shealy. The following is an excerpt from one of her books:

> "Positive and negative experiences register a memory in cell tissue as well as in the energy field. As neurobiologist Dr. Candace Pert has proven, neuro-peptides, *the chemicals triggered by emotions are thoughts converted into matter. Our emotions reside physically in our bodies and interact with our cells and tissues.* In fact, Dr. Pert can no longer separate the mind from the body, she says, because the same kinds of cells that manufacture and receive emotional chemistry in the brain are present throughout the body. Sometimes the body responds emotionally and manufactures emotional chemicals even before the brain has registered a problem. Remember, for instance, how quickly your body reacts to a loud noise before you have had time to think."

What she is saying is very clear yet hardly recognized by modern medicine. Ms. Myss, with Dr. Perts' scientific confirmation, is saying that our emotions become part of our physical matter! Our emotions are not only affecting our cells but becoming part of them.

Norman Cousins author of the book *Anatomy of an Illness* cured himself of a crippling and life-threatening disease.

His experience reinforced some of his deepest beliefs and convictions concerning the nature of the human being. Stricken with a crippling and life-threatening collagen disease, Mr. Cousins regime was based on using laughter as his medicine. He was a huge fan of the Marx brothers and used their movies as medicine. All in consultation and partnership with his often skeptical physicians. He chronicled his recovery in the best-selling *Anatomy of an Illness as Perceived by the Patient: Reflections on Healing and Regeneration*, published in 1979. In the book, generalizing from his own experience and research, he states that "the life force may be the least understood force on earth. Human beings are not locked into fixed limitations. The quest for perfectibility is not a presumption or a blasphemy but the highest manifestation of a great design."

Stress and your brain.

Stress is an emotional fact of life. Every adult has it and it is not by itself a negative thing. It is stressful to raise a family, run a business or please your boss. However, undue or unnecessary stress can be extremely harmful and dis-ease producing if you do not control it and you allow your life to be altered by it. Some people can handle stress and not let it affect their diet, sleep patterns, eating habits or daily rituals. Others allow stress to throw their lives into turmoil. Eating poorly, sleeping less, drinking more etc.

If you are not handling your daily stress it can manifest itself physically and create serious problems. Exercise, meditation and any artistic endeavor can relieve stress.

The amygdala is a part of the brain that is triggered by emotion. It responds to very strong emotions whether positive or negative. Any passionate desire will be burned into the hippocampus part of the brain by the amygdala. Your desire to achieve that goal will become constant. The hippocampus holds that memory at the forefront of your brain and its memory banks. You will be constantly aware of your desired wish. That's why any passionate desire is so effective.

At the same time if an undue amount of stress is involved you may have some problems. The hippocampus is actually damaged by too much stress. The dendrites, tree-like receptors used to communicate with other brain cells (neurons) lose their ability to function.

$\sim$

Bruce McEwen of the Rockefeller University's neuroscience laboratories studied the brain cells of stressed mice. He discovered that the dendrites of the mice were both fewer and shorter as a result of repeated stress. Due to such shrinkage, the hippocampus cells would receive far less information than normally.

McEwen found the opposite in the amygdala (the portion of your brain that regulates emotion.) Chronic stress actually causes the neurons in the amygdala to *grow* and become *more* active. This is not a good thing.

As the amygdala grows you will experience more instability, fear, anger and "generalized anxiety." Generalized anxiety being that state where there is a nonspecific, vague feeling that something is wrong without knowing specifically what that might be. While the hippocampus shrinks, its ability to function decreases along with the ability to match these emotions to specific causes.

All of these findings can be seen on MRI images. McEwen says *"you can actually measure the altered volume of the hippocampus in disorders like major depressive illness."*

How interesting that there is actually a quantifiable, physical damage caused by stress. Remember that the emotions actually become part of our physical makeup (according to Dr. Pert). An overgrown amygdala of an over stressed brain is causing generalized anxiety. This generalized anxiety will then cause our bodies severe damage.

Obviously, you must work to reduce or eliminate harmful stress. Exercise, laughter and creative endeavors are all very effective stress-reducers. Also putting your attention on another who needs your help is a very effective way to reduce stress. You also must stop being in love with the way you presently think and feel. Notice that there is a part of you that enjoys the unnecessary suffering, confusion, and drama that you create.

Your difficulties may seem to be great and you may want to insist that they are harder or more substantial difficulties than the rest of the world's troubles. There are thousands if not millions who would gladly switch circumstances with you in a second. If you are insistent on your present way of thinking and feeling, your chance for recovery is limited. The world isn't impossible. You are. Once I saw this for myself, that I was the cause of my hardship, everything began to change. See this for yourself.

Essentials for Recovery

Desire and Belief

You need 3 strong reasons why you need to get better. Then have a clearly defined goal and a time frame in which to achieve. You need to be quite specific about HOW you will know or measure when you have reached your goal. Write all of this down.

You must not only want to get well you must **believe** you can and begin to ACT AS IF the healing has already begun. Never mind any of the mechanical doubting thoughts and attitudes. Tell them to shut up. You are now too busy healing to listen to them.

A useful affirmation: I AM WELL. Notice not to say I am going to be well or I *will* be well as that puts the healing in the future. The future is not here. I **AM** Well. I **AM** healthy. State your affirmation in the **present tense**. Say these things out loud and MEAN it. The tone and resonance of your voice are creating a vibration that is felt throughout every cell in your body.

Play with which word you put the emphasis on. I am well . . . i AM well . . . i am WELL. Or emphasize all three. **I AM WELL.** Believe what you are giving voice to. Say this and other affirmations as many times a day as you can. Make it a mantra that will begin to burn different pathways and make new connections between the neurons in your brain and your body. Through affirmation, you are imposing your will on the mind and body.

ACT AS IF – One of the most powerful tools for transformation. No matter what your ailment, act like you are healthy. Stand or sit in postures of a healthy vibrant person. Speak in tones that evoke confidence and self-assurance. Think the thoughts you would think, feel the emotions you would feel, say the words you would say if healed. Completely take on the character of someone who has a healthy vibrant body now. You may feel strange doing this at first, but as the days and weeks roll on you will have adapted an entirely different way of thinking and feeling. Not only will your mind be different, but you will body chemistry will have changed.

Take time to close your eyes and visualize your ultimate healthy self. Make the visualization in color and give it motion. After a while of watching your incredible healthy self move around, step into that body and BECOME your healthy self. Feel your strong heartbeat and your powerful body move. Feel the feelings and emotions of a young, healthy, vibrant person. See what you might see in such a state speak how you might speak and be grateful for what you are experiencing. The more time you can spend in these heightened states the better you will begin to feel. Feeling better is guaranteed and has only to do with how sincere you are in your approach.

If you are saying to yourself "this is silly' and "it won't work for me" you have got to adjust your attitude. If you want to do the impossible you have to be willing to go to places in yourself that you are extremely uncomfortable with.

Stay inspired. Read stories that uplift and inspire, surround yourself with those you admire. Avoid negativity in all of its forms be it people, movies, magazines, newspapers, television, gossip, etc. Refuse any thought that is not going to aid you in your recovery. AFFIRMING THOUGHTS ONLY. Surround yourself with beauty. LISTEN TO INSPIRING MUSIC.

Stop poisoning the body and do your best to live according to your natural inclinations and diet. You have all the information you need in this book to do so.

Refuse to get involved in ANY negativity, internally or externally. Notice how the body goes into a panic when thinking certain thoughts and STOP IT. Refuse to indulge yourself in ridiculous fantasies that cause you pain and wreak havoc on your body. You know what I am talking about. The pictures and mental movies we all have about a certain event in your life where you did something foolish, mean or hurtful. Or the opposite of how badly someone treated you and running and re-running the event over and over again in your mind. The fantasies of revenge or looking like the hero in front of your friends or co-workers. The horrible practice of imagining the worst possible scenarios in the future and again putting them on repeat in your brain. Know that ALL of this type of thinking is disease producing. If you pay close attention to your body when you are running these mind films, you will actually FEEL how they are harming you. Stop indulging in this harmful practice. Instead, use your imagination to empower yourself.

CLEAN out your living space. You will be amazed what a relief it is to de-clutter your home and rid yourself of all the accumulated, unnecessary stuff in your home. It is a BIG lift to your spirit to live in a clean orderly house.

Be GRATEFUL. Count your blessings at least twice a day. Preferably when you get up in the morning and when you go to sleep. Write down the things that you are grateful for. I don't care how difficult your situation may be, if you're reading this, you have something to be grateful for. Your eyes must be working fairly well and you are still breathing. Millions of people did not awaken this morning. You did!!!

Get plenty of fresh air and sunshine. Try to be outside for at least 2 hours every day. Get your bare feet in the grass or at least on the Earth. If you are able to move your body do it and do it consistently and as vigorously as you are able. Minimum 20 minutes of exercising every day.

Limit your time in front of the television and computer. Too much screen time is destructive to the body.

If you can only move certain parts of your body, do it. If you are only able to make certain movements make exercises out of them. For instance: Sit in a chair and lift your arms out to the side, slowly and as high as you can. Bring them back down in a controlled fashion and lift them again. Move the limbs with precision and mindfulness like a dancer. Start by doing 10 repetitions five different times. Rest precisely 1 minute between the sets. Work up to doing 25 repetitions then put a lightweight in your hands and go back to 10 reps. Then work up to 25 reps with the weights. Now do that movement to the front and try to make the same improvements. ANY progress you make will prove immensely beneficial.

Of course, this goes for ANY movement you can do. Any movement you are capable of can become an exercise when done with purpose and mindfulness.

Of course, if you are able-bodied you MUST have a regular exercise regime. Fast walking, biking, weight-training, rebounding (mini-trampoline) tai chi, yoga, swimming etc.

Remember your skin is your number one eliminative organ. Sweating is a great way to detoxify the body.

Any kind of resistance training is great, either weight training and/or calisthenics.

The mini-trampoline or rebounder is an excellent form of exercise that will strengthen your entire body and is a great workout for the heart and lungs. You can use a support bar if you are unsteady on your legs. (The Needak brand rebounders are the best I have seen.)

An effective exercise program will increase your confidence, help you to relax, aid your body's eliminative organs, increase your muscle tone, decrease your body fat, increase your heart strength, release endorphins, improve your skin and increase your overall circulation.

If you wish to be healthy you MUST exercise!

Make sure not to over train. This can be dis-ease producing as well. You want to excercise rigorously but you want to avoid repeatedly exhausting your body. A good way to know if you are over-training is to take your resting pulse in the morning when you are well rested. If you are over training your resting pulse rate will be higher than normal on the following day. Also if your muscle soreness is lasting more than two days, if you are having difficulty sleeping, and if you are repeatedly getting injured, you most likely are over training.

Besides a regular excercise regime it is vital to do something creative. Play an instrument, write a story, take an acting class, memorize a great speech, paint a picture. Creativity demands access to other parts of your brain and heart you normally wouldn't be using in your daily life. If you wish to break out of the cycle of disease-producing thoughts and feelings then put yourself in position to have some new and different impressions and access a different part of your brain.

Here are some more suggestions to help turn things around.

- Asking What I Owe vs. Asking What I'm Owed
- Being Grateful vs. Being resentful
- Gaining Understanding vs. Wanting a Quick-fix Solution
- Allowing Solutions vs. Forcing Solutions
- Seeking Contentment vs. Seeking Excitement
- Inwardly Focused vs. Outwardly Focused
- Stubbornness vs. Acceptance
- Do more Listening Less Talking.

GOOD LUCK. HAVE FUN.

10

GIVING BIRTH AND RAISING YOUR HEALTHY CHILD

It is a privilege and a huge responsibility to bring a new life into this world. It is a tremendous opportunity and a very serious undertaking. This is a task that must be done with great consciousness and conscientiousness in order to assure that the child reaches its full potential. In order to see a positive change in the world conscious child rearing and parenting is THE most important matter. Peaceful, intelligent, courageous, emotionally developed and expressive people are the result of parents that practice and value these traits and virtues. By raising a healthy child that is emotionally, intellectually, and physically developed you are giving a gift to the world and to yourself. It takes a lot of Work.

Most people assume they know what they are doing when they become parents. This is an odd phenomenon as being a truly loving and effective parent may be one of the most difficult challenges in life, even to those who are humble and intelligent enough to seek out and accept help. The evidence is clear that most people fail at this endeavor (parenting) as our world is filled with unhappy, miserable, dysfunctional and mentally and physically ill people. These defects are due to poor parenting. How many people can get through the day without some type of mental sedative (prescribed or illicit drugs or alcohol), stimulant or painkilling help? The numbers of those who are not dependent and addicted to drugs are dropping rapidly.

If any sane person with no piloting skills were told to get in the cockpit of a 747 jet and "take it for a spin" they would literally laugh and walk away. Only a crazy person would attempt to fly a jet plane with no idea how to do so. It appears that raising a child may be more difficult and demanding than flying a commercial airliner, so why is it that so many assume they know what they are doing?

Most of Humanity is made up of unconscious people who appear to be awake but are in fact asleep and blind to their shortcomings and inabilities. If you are not dealing with and striving to overcome your deficiencies and limitations as an adult, then having a child is a poor idea. It is even a worse idea if you think you have no deficiencies or limitations.

Just because you can produce a baby does not mean you are equipped to raise the child. Just because you know how your parents raised you does not make you an expert, or even competent as a parent. You would be much better off taking the stance "I have no idea what I am doing, let me find out what this is all about." Questioning the way you were raised is better than mindlessly making all the same mistakes your parents did.

The decision to have a baby ought to come from the most conscientious and broad part of your self. Bringing a new life into this world is a huge responsibility in and of itself. Done with patience, dedication, thoughtfulness, and love it can also be extremely rewarding and a benefit to all mankind. There are millions of infants and children up for adoption. Adoption is a wonderful option as well if you are serious about being a selfless, conscientious parent.

The decision to not have a child can be just as kind-hearted and loving as the decision to have one. Most people have no idea of the time and effort it takes (let alone the money) to raise a child. It is a huge responsibility. If you have any doubts about your ability to be a good parent here is a suggestion. Start by the task of taking care of a plant and after one year if it is still living and healthy you can move on to a pet. If the plant is sick, dying or dead forget about having a pet or a child until you get yourself together. If after one year, the plant is thriving you can move on to a pet. If after two years both the plant and the pet are thriving that is a good sign. If they are not thriving or you have been consistently negligent you can know you have much work to do before you have a child. A plant takes very little mindfulness to keep alive and thriving, just a few minutes a week. A pet takes more time but nowhere near the time you are going to be spending with your child. If taking care of the pet and the plant seems taxing or an unpleasant burden, you may want to opt out of parenthood.

A comedian once said, "I want two kids so I don't have to sit next to strangers on the subway." Having a child for the wrong reasons can be disastrous to all involved and place a greater burden on an already highly burdened society. Here are some of the worst reasons to have a child:

- ꙮ Because that is what I am supposed to do.
- ꙮ To carry on the family name.
- ꙮ To make me proud.
- ꙮ To become a great _____.
- ꙮ So I can have someone to take care of me when I'm old.
- ꙮ So my parents will finally stop nagging me for grandchildren.
- ꙮ So I can collect benefits from the state.
- ꙮ Because that's what my boyfriend/girlfriend wants.
- ꙮ Because that's what my wife/husband wants.
- ꙮ Because I don't want to be the only one in my family/group of friends who don't have a baby.
- ꙮ Because I want a baby.

(Similar to those who "want a puppy" then buy a puppy and realize that they become full grown dogs and less cute and require a lot of love and attention despite the fact they are not so cuddly anymore.) Babies grow up and become teenagers and young adults. You are their Guardian and parent and must have the commitment, knowledge, and energy to raise them responsibly until they can take care of themselves.

Any Parent who abandons and/or neglects their child is doing SEVERE damage to the child, themselves and our world. I believe abandoning your child should be a Crime, here is why:

The statistics concerning children who grow up in single mother homes are staggering. Fatherless children are five times more likely to be criminals, ten times more likely to abuse drugs and twenty times more likely to be imprisoned. Eighty-five percent of youths who are imprisoned grew up without fathers. Children from fatherless homes are five times more likely to commit suicide, nine times more likely to be put in a mental institution, twenty more times more likely to have behavioral disorders. twenty more times as likely to suffer a mental disorder. Thirty-two times more likely to run away from their single parent household.

Seventy-one percent of women who grow up in a single mother home end up getting pregnant while still a teenager, perpetuating this awful circumstance.

Men who grow up fatherless are fourteen times more likely to become rapists.

Eighty percent of rapists come from fatherless homes. TWO parents are essential for a child to develop. Please consider this before making a decision to have a child.

If you happen to be a single mother you can, of course, raise your children successfully but you must make heroic efforts to do so. Find a single mother or two who have raised some children that are healthy, well functioning adults and seek out their guidance continually. Try to find a Father figure for your children, one with high standards and an excellent character.

It also helps to consider the cost of raising a child where you live. Many young parents are often shocked at how much the basic necessities are and what a financial burden exists in raising a child. It is important that you are aware of the average cost of raising a child. Just another reason to get married,

or be in a fully committed relationship before having a child.
Two incomes are better than one.

Reasons to have a child

Both Father and Mother are mutually agreed that they
love each other and want to bring a new life into the
world to increase the joy and harmony on the planet and
to lessen the suffering of the world. They are both willing to take full responsibility and commit to their roles
as guardians and work as hard as they can to give the
child the optimum care, love, and attention until the child
becomes self-sufficient. The parents are responsible for
providing the necessary nurturing, highest moral standards, finest nutrition, and the best education they can
impart to any and all children they bring into this world.
If you are both that willing and committed to parenting
then have a LOT of children because that is exactly what
the world needs.

Poor parenting and inadequate guardianship is the
reason there is so much pain, confusion, and violence
in the world today. The majority of human beings are
producing confused, uneducated, brainwashed and dysfunctional children who have been disabled mentally and
physically by a lack of a proper education, pharmaceutical
poisoning, a toxic diet, mass hypnosis and poor upbring-
ing. These children whose minds and bodies have been
taken over by "modern medicine," the warped media and
hypnotized by television programming and a pop culture
that is almost completely devoid of substance cannot be

anything but a burden on our society. Many have been raised on a poor diet and many are already hooked for life on pharmaceutical drugs. Most children are physically unfit with no education or discipline in that arena. Most children have had their ability to reason and think for themselves severely handicapped and are unequipped and disinterested in questioning the things they have been taught. Most of the popular music, movies, and TV shows are aimed at keeping the masses ignorant and easily controlled (read *The Tavistock Institute* by Daniel Estulin.)

If you decide not to have a child it would be wise to educate yourself about natural birth control as birth control pills are very dangerous and sometimes deadly.

Birth control

Birth control pills are extremely damaging to your health and should be avoided at all costs. If you have ever taken them I would suggest waiting at least one year before trying to get pregnant.

I know millions of women take these pills and believe them to be relatively safe. They are not. Let's take a look at one of the more popular birth control pills sold recently.

It is called "Yaz." The following are listed as "side effects." These "side effects" are common among most birth control pills.

"SIDE EFFECTS: Nausea, vomiting, headache, bloating, breast tenderness, swelling of the ankles/feet

(fluid retention), or weight change may occur. Vaginal bleeding between periods (spotting) or missed/irregular periods may occur, especially during the first few months of use. If any of these effects persist or worsen, notify your doctor promptly. If you miss 2 periods in a row (or 1 period if the pill has not been used properly), contact your doctor for a pregnancy test.

Remember that your doctor has prescribed this medication because he or she has judged that the benefit to you is greater than the risk of side effects. Many people using this medication do not have serious side effects.

Tell your doctor right away if any of these serious side effects occur: unusual changes in vaginal bleeding (such as continuous spotting, sudden heavy bleeding, missed periods).

This medication may rarely cause serious (sometimes fatal) problems from blood clots (such as deep vein thrombosis, pulmonary embolism, stroke, heart attack). Talk to your doctor about the risks and benefits of this birth control pill. Get medical help right away if you experience: sudden shortness of breath, chest/jaw/left arm pain, unusual sweating, confusion, coughing up blood, sudden dizziness/fainting, pain/swelling/warmth in the groin/calf, tingling/weakness/numbness in the arms/legs, unusual headaches (including headaches with vision changes/lack of coordination, worsening of migraines, sudden/very severe headaches), slurred speech, weakness on one side of the body, sudden vision changes (such as partial/complete blindness).

Get medical help right away if any of these rare but serious side effects occur: lumps in the breast, severe stomach/abdominal pain, dark urine, yellowing eyes/ skin, mental/mood changes (such as new/worsening depression, suicidal thoughts).

A very serious allergic reaction to this drug is rare. However, get medical help right away if you notice any symptoms of a serious allergic reaction, including: rash, itching/swelling (especially of the face/tongue/ throat), severe dizziness, trouble breathing.

This is not a complete list of possible side effects. If you notice other effects not listed above, contact your doctor or pharmacist."

This is a common example of listed side effects for many birth control pills.

The drug company presented a TV commercial showing young, energetic and euphoric women pushing, punching and kicking CGI words (commonly related to side effects of other birth control pills) such as 'irritability", "nausea," "severe cramping,""increased anxiety" and "bloating." I guess the advertisers forgot to have these actresses punch or kick the word "stroke," "heart attack" and sometimes "fatal blood clots." Scores of deaths and strokes have been caused by this drug (and many other birth control pills) and there are lawsuits piled up against the manufacturer. The commercial would end up being much longer if the actresses had to kick and punch ALL the "side effects" listed above.

This is one example of many birth control pills on the market. You should know that ALL birth control pills are extremely dangerous and cause severe adverse health effects. The attempt to chemically suppress your body's natural cycles, shut down and/or redirect your hormones is an unintelligent and horrible idea that will only wreak havoc in your body. Weight gain, severe acne and headaches are common.

If you have never taken them do not start. There are other safe effective ways of birth control that do not include damaging your body at all. There are natural ways to know when you are fertile and when you are not. When you have an understanding of your natural cycle you will then know the prime time to try to get pregnant as well as when you are infertile.

I suggest a book called *Taking Charge of your Fertility* by Toni Weschler. This book is also very helpful to couples that are trying to conceive a child as well as for those who want to avoid pregnancy by natural means. You will learn by different methods to know when you are fertile and when you are not, without having to subject yourself to these dangerous and sometimes deadly pills.

Here are some added reasons to get married before you have a child. According to the Brookings Institute;

> "Since 1970, out-of-wedlock birth rates have soared. In 1965, 24 percent of black infants and 3.1 percent of white infants were born to single mothers. By 1990 the rates had risen to 64 percent for black infants, 18 percent for whites. Every year about one million more children are born into fatherless families. If we have learned any policy lesson well over the past 25 years, it is that for children living in single-parent homes,

the odds of living in poverty are great. The policy implications of the increase in out-of-wedlock births are staggering."

According to the Brookings Institute: "There are three rules you need to fulfill as a person to avoid poverty: Finish high school, get a job do not have a baby before you get married." "Seventy-five percent of those who have done these three things have joined the middle class . . . only 2% live in poverty."

General care of the child

IF you decide to have a child: *It is your responsibility to keep yourself healthy and fit during your pregnancy.*

It is the parent's job, especially the mother, to be as healthy and fit as she can be. Gaining weight from your pregnancy is natural, but being overweight or carrying excess fat is unhealthy, unnatural and creates a huge strain on the mother and the child. It might be "normal" in our twisted culture but there is absolutely nothing "natural" about it.

To have a healthy child it is necessary to have already established healthy eating habits before you are pregnant. Obviously, raw organic fruits, vegetables, seeds, and nuts are the best way to feed yourself. Eating according to your biology will give you and your baby the best chance at having a truly successful, safe, healthy pregnancy and a healthy, sound child. If 100% raw is too much for you do at LEAST 75% raw while pregnant and avoid all animal products.

If you have any concern that you may need a special diet now that you are pregnant . . . you don't. Millions of animals in nature are born every day and NONE of them move away from their natural diet (which is without question entirely raw food). No matter what your doctor or any other salesman says, this is the truth. You are pregnant. You DO NOT have a disease that needs "treatment."

Exercise is essential to your well-being and necessary for a successful pregnancy and birth. It should be a part of your daily routine. You can exercise right up until the day you give birth. Doing so will allow you to give birth more easily and recovery from the birth more quickly. It will also allow you to deal with a lot of the physical changes that occur during pregnancy along with the significant changes in your hormonal balance. Exercise significantly lowers your stress levels. Exercise releases endorphins. Exercise will also increase your body's abilities to deal with pain and give you extra confidence in your physical abilities. Exercise oxygenates your bloodstream, thus your growing baby will have more oxygen in the womb. Exercise will help you clear your mind and relax. This will benefit you and your baby.

There are endless choices of exercise regimes for the pregnant woman. I recommend weight training and/or calisthenics for strength training and a good stretching or yoga routine along with some cardiovascular exercise such as biking, fast walking, Stairmaster or elliptical trainer. (Jogging is NOT a good exercise.) Stick with low impact exercises. Make a commitment to increase your strength, flexibility, and endurance before giving birth. Being fit and strong will not only make the actual birth easier, it will help you recover very quickly.

In order to have a truly healthy baby the mother must avoid all the common poisons such as dairy products, cigarette smoke, meat, processed foods, pharmaceutical drugs, illicit drugs, caffeine, alcohol, pesticides, fluoride (found in tap water and toothpaste), aluminum in anti-perspirants, salt, chlorine (found in tap water), processed sugar, refined sugar, processed foods and vaccines, strong electromagnetic fields, as well as toxins in the home such as toxic cleaning products, glues and aluminum pots and pans (cast iron is the safest).

If you have had a history of using drugs prescribed, illicit or commonly used (caffeine, nicotine, painkillers) you should do a long cleanse until your body is completely rid of them. That means ALL drugs. Your body does not know the difference between a prescribed drug and an "illicit" drug or a "legal" drug or "illegal" drug. THE FACT IS ALL DRUGS ARE POISONOUS AND CAN HARM YOUR BABY. Marijuana which after years of man-made hybridization now has extremely high levels of THC. According to a 2012 literature review published in Clinical Lactation, babies that have been exposed to THC through breast milk reportedly have increased the risk of experiencing the following:

- ✐ Increased tremor
- ✐ Poor sucking reflex
- ✐ Decreased feeding time
- ✐ Slow weight gain
- ✐ Changes in visual responses
- ✐ Delayed motor development

(Check the Fasting chapter for more guidance on cleaning out your body.)

Alcohol

When you drink alcohol while pregnant so does your baby. Alcohol passes right through the placenta into the fetus. The alcohol that you drink passes through your bloodstream relatively quickly, yet it lingers in your baby's bloodstream a very long time and does irreparable harm to your baby's brain and central nervous system causing mild and/or serious birth defects that are irreversible.

Obviously, if you have an addiction to alcohol you must not get pregnant as you will be subjecting your child to horrible circumstances.

Alcohol is the cause of a lot of pain and anguish on so many different levels. Many people use alcohol to self-medicate and dull the emotional pain they are living in. Facing your problems and dealing with your emotions is the ONLY real solution. "Drinking your pain away" only increases your pain and will destroy your family. Be Intelligent and avoid alcohol whether you are pregnant or not.

Also, negative emotions and stress can cause toxicity in the bloodstream. Do your best to stay calm and centered. I highly recommend that you make Meditation a part of your daily ritual in the morning and evening. (Read Thich Nhat Hanh's *The Miracle of Mindfulness*.)

Remember that your body is the soil you will be using to grow your child. Do all you can to make sure it is

rid of poisons. Also, you must do your best to stay emotionally calm and relaxed leading up to and during your
nine months of pregnancy. By doing this you will avoid
MANY problems that most mothers and babies have to
deal with and be able to give birth to a Truly Healthy
child.

Giving birth

The birth process is a crucial part of human life. There
is a specific order and design built into the natural birth
process that protects and insures both the mother and
the baby's well-being and health. Every aspect of the natural birthing process is quintessential. Any interference
will only do harm. The more interference, the more harm.
The birthing process carries with it a highly intelligent
design that ought to be revered, respected and unob-
structed. Human babies are born helpless. The parents
must be very capable, attentive and willing. The baby
is leaving behind a very familiar, quiet and comfortable
world of warm water and mostly darkness to a world of
cool air, loud sounds and bright light. It is a shocking
experience. Similar to what we experience when we dive
into a pool of cold water.

All of a sudden the infant's entire world changes, air
must be breathed by the lungs that have been unused up
until birth and are now essential for life. Food must be
taken through the mouth instead of the umbilical cord,
and a sea of air is the new environment. All incredibly
momentous changes along with the obvious fact that

there is a whole new set of visual, auditory and kines-
thetic stimulus. The more aware you are of this as a
parent and the more you work to help your child make
this transition smoothly the healthier and sounder your
child will be. As a parent/guardian it is your responsibility to make this transition as comfortable and safe as
possible. By doing so you enhance the possibilities of the
child tremendously. The child will feel your efforts and be
extremely comforted.

Unfortunately when doctors and hospitals are
involved this transition often becomes disastrous. Doctors
tend to treat pregnancy like a disease and childbirth like
a catastrophe . . . often creating just that. They perform
all sorts of crazy, counter-intuitive and dangerous treatments to the mother and unborn baby. These senseless
acts are damaging to the child's physical, emotional and
mental well being and you need to protect you and your
baby from them.

Dr. Robert Mendelsohn, who practiced medicine for
30 years, once said: "when you are pregnant go to your
doctor, listen to everything he has to say then go home
and do the exact opposite." I know these days there are
some doctors that have real intelligence and understand
that pregnancy is not a disease and that childbirth is
the most natural of all human processes. Do your best
to seek out a doctor with this non-invasive, natural type
of approach. They do exist and are a huge bonus to our
world. If you cannot find one like that, just hire a midwife
and a doula.

Animals and humans in nature have been, and are
giving birth all over the world for thousands of centuries

right up to today without ANY "aid" from doctors, epidurals, amniocentesis, vaccines, ultrasounds, vitamin shots, antibiotics, drugs or hospitals. Most mammals seek out dark, quiet places to give birth. They usually are alone. Can anyone argue that this is natural? In a hospital the delivering mother is usually put in a loud extremely bright room, filled with noisy machinery, a large and toxic electromagnetic field, placed on her back (to make it easier for the doctors) which is NOT the best birth position for most mothers, with a bunch of strangers walking around in masks and wearing latex gloves . . . scary enough for an adult but just think how shocking and strange it must be for a newborn infant.

If a cesarean birth is deemed "necessary," (most of them are NOT necessary) the natural birth process will be unnecessarily and violently interrupted by a sharp knife ripped across the muscles of the mother's abdomen to release the baby from the womb before it is properly born and both the mother and child will suffer the repercussions of such an unnatural birth. The mother obviously will be given high doses of pain medication, which of course ends up in the breast milk she will soon be feeding the baby. This will damage the mother and the baby's health.

Effects of unnatural birth

Doctors and hospitals make more money with a cesarean birth and it is convenient for them. It is also very convenient for them to make an appointment for your baby's birth. They often tell the birthing mother that the "baby is breached" or "the umbilical cord is wrapped around the baby's neck so we have to do a cesarean." Both of these situations are quite common and can be easily corrected by a skilled midwife or doula. More and more doctors are simply using cesareans as a convenience to keep their schedule intact. An embarrassing fact that places you and your baby in peril. Here are some facts you should know concerning this issue of Cesarean births:

Soc Sci Med. 1993 Nov; 37(10):1177–98. Sakala C. Pub Med.gov:

> Between 1965 and 1986, the United States cesarean section rate increased from 4.5 to 24.1%. Increasingly, childbearing women and their advocates, along with many others, have recognized that a large proportion of cesareans confers a broad array of risks without providing any medical benefit. A growing literature examines the diverse causes of medically unnecessary cesareans and the diverse effects of surgical birth on women, infants, and families. Various programs and policies have been proposed or implemented to reduce cesarean rates. In recent decades, many other nations have also experienced a sharply escalating cesarean section rate. It is reasonable to conclude that a largely uncontrolled international pandemic of medically unnecessary cesarean births is occurring.

From The Public Citizen May 1994:

According to the National Center for Health Statistics (NCHS), the c-section rate nationwide increased more than four-fold in a little less than 20 years, rising from 5.5 percent in 1970 to 24.7 percent in 1988. Since then the rate has varied only slightly, actually decreasing modestly after 1990. Meanwhile, between 1985 and 1992, the VBAC rate (the proportion of women with a previous c-section who deliver vaginally) has steadily risen from 6.6 to 25.4 percent. Our own data, collected mainly from state vital records offices, show a nationwide cesarean rate of 22.6 percent for 1992.

—From *Live Science*: Amber Angelle |
    November 21, 2010

Between 1996 and 2007, the number of C-sections performed in U.S. hospitals rose by more than 50 percent to an all-time high: Almost one in three *pregnant women*, regardless of race or ethnicity, now delivers via a cesarean section, according to the Centers for Disease Control and Prevention.

Please do not subject yourself and your baby to this unnecessary and harmful operation. Speak to your midwife and doula. Read all you can about natural childbirth including the books mentioned and listed at the end of this chapter. It is a very rare occasion when this operation is actually necessary. Besides unnecessary procedures like cesareans, at times barbaric tools are used to "assist" in the birth along with painkillers that damage the baby's brain and deaden the mother's ability to respond to the helpless infant while poisoning her breast milk.

Amniocentesis is another medical invention that is supposed to tell you if your child will have any birth defects. It is close to useless and can be very dangerous. It makes NO sense to stick an 8 to 10 inch needle into the mother's womb, so close to a developing infant.

The fact is that a hospital is the antithesis of a natural birthplace or a safe one.

Besides the glaring lights, lack of fresh air, electromagnetic fields masked strangers, beeping heart monitors and unnatural settings the baby's birth is greatly hampered by absurd medical rituals and the birth becomes extremely difficult. Drugs designed to kill pain shut down key neuro-pathways needed for a healthy birth. These drugs ingested by the mother poison the baby while breastfeeding causing serious health problems immediately and/or in the future.

New-born babies are given painful mandatory shots and vaccines filled with poisons then carted off to a nursery or incubator to complete isolation in a plastic box, so the mother can "rest." This is absurd, as the mother and child will be nothing but alarmed, agitated, nervous and depressed that they are not together. The Mother and Child need to stay together, preferably skin to skin for as long and often as possible. Resting will not be possible due to the instinctual agitation of being separated. This is highly unnatural and very damaging emotionally and physically to both mother and child. If you need any convincing of this, try taking ANY mammals offspring away from them right after birth and you will end up badly injured. Animals have their instincts intact. Humans have had most of them removed by social programming.

Circumcision

Newborn male babies commonly have the tip of their penis cut off with no anesthesia or effort to dull the excruciating pain. This barbaric, harmful, useless and "accepted" practice is called "circumcision." It ought to be called what it is, infant torture and infant mutilation. No matter what your religious, social or medical beliefs might be, cutting off the tip of your baby's penis is objectively cruel, inhumane and should be deemed a crime. It is so traumatizing to the child that they often pass out from the pain. You must protect your child from this barbarism. Would you allow your daughter to be mutilated? Of course not, so why allow your son to be mutilated?

What kind of an impression would it leave on you if you visited another country and the first thing your hosts did was cut off a part of your penis? The part of the body with the most nerve endings? Well your baby is coming from a very peaceful, cozy, intimate world and then right after birth is delivered into a whole new world and one of its first impressions is this extremely violent and painful mutilation. There is no way that this mutilation can be helpful to the child. It can ONLY do harm physically, mentally and emotionally. As a parent, you must protect your child from this atrocity. Any medical explanation of why it is done is a façade for the real reason it is done. More profits for the hospital. Any religious belief advocating this type of torture is archaic, barbaric, ignorant and Very cruel. The Creator made no mistake creating a foreskin. You and all religious leaders and doctors who condone this have made a grave mistake believing in this mutilation ritual. Why not allow your son to grow to an age where he can make a conscious well-informed decision for himself and if he chooses to cut this part of his body off (sounds absurd doesn't it?) then he can proceed to have a full understanding of the mutilation (with pain-killers) and its effects, instead of torturing a young, helpless infant because of something you "believe?" If your religious text told you to gauge your baby's eye out, would you do it?

Ultrasound

This procedure is commonly done and viewed by the general public as benign and safe. According to many scientists and doctors, they are not safe. Ultrasounds raise the temperature of anything the wand is pointed towards. We know that when an adult human being has a temperature of over 104 degrees (F) that it is very dangerous and could even be fatal. That is about 5 Degrees above the average human temperature which is 98.6 degrees. Ultrasound can easily cause increases of 5 degrees or more especially if used by a poorly trained operator. Imagine a fetus still forming in the womb with only a thin layer of skull to protect it's forming brain and nervous system and it gets bombarded with that kind of intense heat. Obviously, that can and will do damage.

From the FDA in 2004: "Ultrasound is a form of energy, and even at low levels, laboratory studies have shown it can produce physical effect in tissue, such as jarring vibrations and a rise in temperature." This is consistent with research conducted in 2001 in which an ultrasound transducer aimed directly at a miniature hydrophone placed in a woman's uterus recorded sound "as loud as a subway train coming into the station."

Electromagnetic fields

We live in a world where we are constantly being bombarded by radio frequencies and electromagnetic fields. These radiations can create a myriad of health problems including cancer, tumors, depression, insomnia and other symptoms as well. Make sure that your home and your infant's bedroom is free of these high levels of EMFs. If you are using a baby monitor make sure it is NOT a wireless one as they have very high output of these EMFs. You can buy a baby monitor that has a wire, they emit much less EMFs. If you have a wireless router you or your baby should be at least 15 feet away from it at all times as these routers emit very strong radiations. Do your family a favor and get a wired router.

The highest radiations in normal home life are the wireless router, the back of your refrigerator and a microwave oven. Frankly, there is NO reason to have a microwave oven as microwaves destroy any food you place inside of it. If you live in an apartment or multi-family dwelling make sure that you know where your neighbor's refrigerators are placed as the EMF easily pass through sheetrock walls. Keep yourself and your child at least 10–12 feet away from the wireless router at all times and/or just turn it off when not in use. Wired routers emit much less radiation. These radiations easily penetrate walls so make sure you keep a good distance from these appliances.

Many homes have now been outfitted with "smart" meters from the utility companies that can send information about your electricity usage straight to the company. However convenient that maybe it also has created a major problem for home-owners as the EMF's radiating from these machines are extremely high and many have reported that they are creating serious health problems. There are companies that actually sell devices you can put around these meters that block most of the harmful radiations.

If you want to get accurate measurements of the EMF's around your house you can buy a Trifield Meter model 100xe.

Never put laptops on your lap. Keep them and your desktop computer at least seven inches away from your head and vital organs. You can buy a lap shield to deflect the radiation from your body if you insist on placing the computer on your lap.

Vaccines

According to Dr. Doreen Granpeesheh, founder of the Center for Autism and Related Disorders:

In 1978 the prevalence of Autism was 1 in 15,000 children. In 1995 it was 1 in 500. In 2005 it was 1 in 150. In 2010, 1 in 110. And the rate of Autism continues to climb. In fact, according to National Health Center for Health Statistics in 2016 this rate has drastically climbed to an alarming 1 in 36 children diagnosed with autism. Yet the mainstream media remains silent on the issue.

If you read the previous chapter, The Myth of Contagion, you know very clearly how this author views the idea of vaccination. The idea that vaccines "protect your health" is as absurd as the idea that chimpanzees would make good pilots. I would never allow my loved ones to ride in a plane piloted by chimps and I would never allow them to be vaccinated as well.

Babies born in hospitals are subjected to these deadly disease-producing vaccines. These vaccines contain toxic chemicals, including mercury, formaldehyde, aluminum, MSG, remains from aborted fetuses, benzethonium chloride and derivatives of human tissue. A new toxic substance has recently been detected in vaccines: Glyphosate—the active ingredient in Monsanto's deadly herbicide Roundup. If you think that any of these items will create health or "protect" your child, you have been brainwashed. There are thousands and thousands of cases where parents have reported severe and harmful effects of these vaccines immediately following the injections including, fevers, nausea, stroke, facial deformities, toxic shock, allergies, brain damage, autism, nervous system damage, and death.

If you think a vaccine has ever helped anybody or prevented or stopped any disease or epidemics you have

believed in the smoke and mirrors charade the pharmaceutical companies and their bought off media have
concocted. Take a look at your next "news" cast and notice
that 50% to 70% of the commercials are for the major
Drug Companies. If you think that is not a conflict of
interests you need to think some more. Vaccinations and
their statistics are easily manipulated and adjusted to
present the illusory picture that it is intended to show,
just how "miraculous" they are. If you take the time to
understand that the symptoms of any disease can be easily
manipulated and "officially" altered by the CDC, DOH,
NIH, Drug Companies and their partners in crime the
media, you will begin to understand how easy it is to
make vaccines appear like they are effective or "working."

Because the very people who create and "treat" dis-
ease are working together to earn billions in profits the
amount of deception is endless. Any disease can conveniently be "eradicated" by simply giving it a different
name. All that needs to be done is to "officially" change
the diagnostic criteria from one day to the next, which
DOES happen, the illusion of a disease being "eradicated"
or "cured" is produced. The disease has in fact not been
eradicated by a "miracle drug" but has been eradicated by
simply by changing the name of the disease or the symptoms used to define the disease. If for instance, you have
a disease called Polio and the health authorities decide
to one day call it Spinal Meningitis, after a year of poisonous vaccines (that admittedly kill and maim scores
of children) the illusion is created that the Polio disease
has been "eradicated" by the vaccine. But that is not the
truth. Or if you simply change the diagnostic criteria to

no longer include major symptoms the same illusion is created. You can also have your clinics, hospitals, doctors and media partners stop reporting cases. It is THAT simple. "Vaccines saved the day," says the media but the fact is vaccines do not save or have ever saved anyone. It is only an illusion, a lie.

If you think events like this aren't constantly going on in the pharmaceutical world and media then you are living with your head in the sand.

Of course Pharmaceutical companies "lobby" (a euphemism for bribery) congressmen and senators to push through legislation making all these vile vaccine concoctions mandatory for your children and now for adults. But the US Constitution clearly states that you are free to practice your religion and many religious people and others have asserted their rights to refuse vaccination. Of course, this is a huge threat to the multi-billion dollar vaccine machine and they are working every day to take your freedom of choice away from you through massive disinformation programs, fear mongering, bribery and lies. Doctors who are against vaccination and support their patients right to decline are often vehemently denounced and persecuted by the AMA. The people who run the world want you to be sick and in need of medical care. Vaccinations are a sure way of getting that result. The fact is vaccines do not prevent anything . . . but health. They do create a lot of disease and death.

Back on September 23, 2014, an Italian court in Milan granted compensation to a boy for the autism he suffered as a result of a vaccine. A childhood vaccine against six childhood diseases caused the boy's permanent autism and brain damage. While the Italian press has covered this story extensively and has considered it's public health implications in open forums, the U.S. media has blacked out the story completely.

Each year HMO plans give doctors several thousand dollars in bonuses. One of the requirements for a patient's chart to pass the test is that they are "fully vaccinated."

According to the CDC website budget, The 2015 fiscal budget of the CDC is $6.6 billion, a decrease of $243 million from 2014. However, "Vaccines for Children" is the largest category within the budget, and it increased from $3.5 billion in 2014 to $4 billion in 2015, an increase of $514 million. So the American taxpayer, through the CDC, is forcibly purchasing $4 billion of vaccines from the pharmaceutical industry. It has been my experience that the greater the amount of money involved the greater the amount of crime and deception. Big Pharma wants you and your kids ALL hooked on their drugs and they are willing to pay for it.

From Global Research:

> "Though the US contains just 5% of the world population, it consumes over half of all pre-scribed medication and a phenomenal *80% of the world's supply of painkillers.* Those who admit to taking prescription drugs on average take four different prescription drugs daily. Taking mas-sive amounts of prescription drugs has caused an epidemic that's part of a sinister plan to squeeze yet more profit out of a system designed to keep humans chronically unhealthy.

Even more alarming is the fact that death by medical error at near a quarter million people annually has become the *third largest killer* of US citizens behind heart disease and cancer. Other more recent studies have estimated upwards of up to 440,000 *have died yearly* from preventable mistakes at hospitals. Blind obedience to Big Pharma and a conventional medical system too dependent on surgery and technology has inflicted more harm than good on the U.S. population."

I imagine there are some decent, well-intentioned employees at the CDC but as a whole, the CDC along with other government agencies cares very little about the health of you and your family. The CDC, FDA, NIH, HHS, along with the drug companies, are so wrought with fraud, corruption and crime they make the Mafia look good. Many doctors and government workers are paid ridiculous salaries by pharmaceutical companies to "work" for their companies for a year or two, knowing full well their skills are not worth the millions they are getting paid in salary. However these companies and their now wealthy "employees" will realize their value once their cushy jobs end and they go back to work for the FDA, CDC (or other agencies) to determine what drugs will be "approved" and which ones will not. This conflict of interest absurdity has been going on for decades.

There are no warranties or guarantees of efficacy safety made by the drug companies who make these vaccines. How strange. Almost all manufacturers of safety products stand behind their goods with guarantees and warranties, yet NOT ONE drug company guarantees ANYTHING about these substances that go into your child's bloodstream. Drug companies will even admit that your child may still get the disease they are supposedly being vaccinated against!

As of 1986 drug companies will never pay another dime out of their coffers in court for lawsuits by those they have injured, disabled or to the families of those they kill. Thanks to the passing of National Childhood Vaccine Injury Act (it does SOUND as if it is FOR the victims but it is exactly the opposite) There now exists a ceiling of $250,000.00 in damages for those who are injured and are able to win a lawsuit (a very difficult task) against the drug companies. It costs 3 Million dollars to care for an autistic person for their lifetime. $250,000.00 is not fair at all, especially considering that massive profits drug companies rake in each year.

Does that money paid from lost suits come out of Big Pharma's pockets? Nope. It comes out of your pocket as each vaccine sold now has an added tax that is collected and deposited and placed in a fund to pay for lost lawsuits for damages and death inflicted on the populace. If vaccines are harmless and actually work why don't the drug companies stand behind them with guarantees? Why did they have to bribe government officials to pass a law that gives them complete immunity in a court of law? The answer is simple. The lawsuits would destroy their companies and they know it.

The following from Barbara Loe Fisher:

"On Nov. 14, 1986, President Ronald Reagan signed the National Childhood Vaccine Injury Act of 1986 into law, instituting first-time vaccine safety reforms in the U.S. vaccination system and creating the first no-fault federal vaccine injury compensation program alternative to a lawsuit against vaccine manufacturers and pediatricians. Twenty-two years later, on Nov. 18, 2008, I made a statement to the Advisory Commission on Childhood Vaccines (ACCV) and questioned whether the compensation program is fatally flawed and so broken that it should be repealed. Many parents are wondering whether it would be better to return to civil court without restrictions to sue vaccine manufacturers and doctors for injuries and deaths their children suffered after receiving federally recommended vaccines."

During its two-decade history, two out of three individuals applying for federal vaccine injury compensation have been turned away empty-handed, even though to date $1.8 billion has been awarded to more than 2,200 plaintiffs out of some 12,000 who have applied. Today, nearly 5,000 vaccine injury claims are sitting in limbo because they represent children who suffered brain and immune system dysfunction after vaccination but have been diagnosed with regressive autism, which is not recognized by the program as a compensable event. There is $2.7 billion sitting in the Trust Fund, which could have been awarded to vaccine victims."

The fact is, vaccines do not prevent anything but health and can only cause harm. Any source that says differently is either brainwashed and/or selling you something.

The drug companies and vaccine salesmen "educate" doctors. That's a fact and any new product or vaccine is marketed and promoted to doctors by salesmen and in many cases, doctors are bribed to dispense a new drug/vaccine by "gifts" (such as luxury vacations, cash rewards or some other consumer product) and other perks.

William W. Thompson, PhD, Senior Scientist with the CDC has stepped forward and admitted the 2004 paper entitled "Age at first measles-mumps-rubella vaccination in children with autism and school-matched control subjects: a population-based study in metropolitan Atlanta," which has been used repeatedly by the CDC to deny the MMR-autism connection, was a FRAUD. http://www.ncbi.nlm.nih.gov/pubmed/14754936

Dr. Thompson has admitted the 340% increase in boys receiving the MMR vaccine "on time," as opposed to delayed, was buried by himself, Dr. DeStefano, Dr. Bhasin, Dr. Yeargin-Allsopp, and Dr. Boyle . . . Dr. Thompson first called and spoke with Dr. Brian Hooker, who then revealed the information to Dr. Andrew Wakefield and the Autism Media Channel.

Dr. Thompson: "I regret that my coauthors and I omitted statistically significant information in our 2004 article published in the journal Pediatrics. The omitted data suggested that African American males who received the MMR vaccine before age 36 months were at increased risk for autism."

On July 29th, 2015, Representative Bill Posey Fla. (R-8th district) called for an investigation of this crime by the CDC. The fact is that whenever you hear the term "Healthcare" you can be sure of two things. Real Health is not involved. Drug distribution and massive profits are.

Recently, the U.S. Department of Justice (DOJ) reported Pfizer using its influential money to bribe foreign governments and their health officials. The apparent goal was to use Pfizer's money to create unfair economic advantages in the market to peddle their pharmaceuticals and vaccines.

Pfizer was caught doing some shady backroom deals in Bulgaria, Croatia, Kazakhstan, and Russia, which violated the Foreign Corrupt Practices Act (FCPA). The DOJ report stated, "Corrupt pay-offs to foreign officials in order to secure lucrative contracts creates an inherently uneven marketplace and puts honest companies at a disadvantage," said Assistant Director McJunkin. "Those that attempt to make these illegal backroom deals to influence contract procurement can expect to be investigated by the FBI and appropriately held responsible for their actions." In this case, it seems the influence-buying pharmaceutical companies get away with being fined only $45 million in fines, which amounts to a financial slap on the wrist. You should know this is not an isolated incident; it's the tip of the proverbial influence-buying iceberg. Bribery from Big Pharma in the United States, however, takes on a more subtle form or "style."

Your pediatrician and family doctor have been "influenced."

Here is the apparently brutal truth: Bribery takes place in the United States in the legal form of "speaking fees," plus your doctor may be on Big Pharma's payroll. Should we consider Congressional lobbying money too?

In 2009 Merck released a 72-page document showing they paid doctors at least $18,810,495.52—close to $19 million—in the third and fourth quarters of that year for medical doctors to speak favorably about their pills and vaccines.[3] Additionally, Pro Repulica's "Dollar for Docs" project shows at least $761.3 million had been paid to doctors across the United States:

Does the U.S. Government do business with criminal companies?

Do the CDC and FDA transact business with companies found guilty and fined for breaking the law? Given Big Pharma's involvement with vaccines and drugs, that is a very relevant question.

Here is what we know that needs to be evaluated in light of the above information about doctors' Big Pharma payouts.

⌒ The CDC recommends at least 3 pneumococcal vaccines for each child before 6 months of age.[1]

1   See the CDC's vaccine price list here:http://www.cdc.gov/vaccines/programs/vfc/cdc-vac-price-list.htm

- ⋄ Pfizer has contract #200-2012-50135 with the CDC[7, 8]
- ⋄ The contract is worth $8,386,013.00, to manufacture the Prevnar 13 (a pneumococcal vaccine)[2]
- ⋄ The vaccine is priced at $102.03 a vaccine.[3, 4]

Of course, the above incident is not isolated to Pfizer alone. You can find similar information on Merck, Sanofi, GlaxoSmithKline, and Novartis — all of whom have contracts with the CDC and have had a presence on the Department of Justice website.

In 2009 Doctors received 18 Million dollars from Merck to promote their toxic vaccines. I repeat that is only for speaking fees. That is only one company.

Julie Gerberding, former head of the Centers for Disease Control, paved the way for eventual approval for Merck's Gardasil vaccine, guaranteeing billions in profits for her future employer. After her stint at the CDC, she became President of the Vaccine Division at Merck Pharmaceuticals. This is a VERY common practice at the FDA, NIH and CDC. It is also a clear and direct conflict of interest—and as I view it, completely unethical. Politicians are frequently approached by drug companies to vote a certain way to increase their profits (no matter how many are killed or disabled by their drugs

---

2   See Pfizer's contract with the CDC here: www.hhs.gov/open/recordsand reports/prevention/solicitations/pediatric_vaccines_071912.pdf

3   See the Department of Justice press release about Pfizer here: http://www.justice.gov/opa/pr/2012/August/12-crm-980.html

4   http://vactruth.com/2010/01/04/julie-gerberding-primed-big-pharmas-pump-with-flu-and-hpv-vaccines/

and vaccines) then once the vote is done the bought off politician will receive a "job" at the drug company along with a huge salary, benefits, and bonuses.

> "A single vaccine given to a six-pound newborn is the equivalent of giving a 180-pound adult 30 vaccinations on the same day. Include the toxic effects of high levels of aluminum and formaldehyde contained in some vaccines, and the synergist toxicity could be increased to unknown levels . . . Bilary transport is the major biochemical route by which mercury is removed from the body, and infants cannot do this very well. They also do not possess the renal (kidney) capacity to remove aluminum. Additionally, mercury is a well-known inhibitor of kidney function."

Boyd Haley PhD., Professor and Chair, Department of Chemistry, University of Kentucky:

> "Some additional ingredients (as listed by the CDC in their website) include antibiotics which you could be allergic to; aluminum which when combined with silicon deficiency results in neurofibrillary tangles seen in Alzheimer's; formaldehyde—a toxic carcinogenic substance used to preserve dead people; MSG—a potent excitotoxin which like aspartame can cause seizures and brain tumours; egg protein to which you could have life-threatening anaphylactic reaction; and sulfites another toxin injected directly

into bloodstream. What the CDC does not admit is that 13 vaccines at present are cultured on aborted fetal tissue (human diploid cells). They also fail to mention the ethyl mercury containing preservative thimerosal which has been the ONLY dangerous substance in vaccines to received mainstream media attention . . ."

Rebecca Carley MD, VIDS Expert, *"Inoculations: The True Weapon of Mass Destruction"*:

"All vaccine ingredients are poisonous, carcinogenic, or potentially harmful to the skin, gastro-intestinal, pulmonary, neurological and immune systems . . . What about formaldehyde? Are we going to wait until another brave physician or scientist writes about the damaging effects of formaldehyde on our children's brains before we are called to demand that formaldehyde be removed? Or about Problems associated with having Polysorbate 80 in the vaccine? Polysorbate-80 is used in pharmacology to assist in the delivery of certain drugs or chemotherapeutic agents across the blood-brain barrier. What bacterial, yeast, heavy metal or other vaccine containing ingredients need to pass into the brains of our children?"

Lawrence B. Palevsky, MD, FAAP, Pediatrician, *Aluminum and Vaccine Ingredients: What Do We Know? What Don't We Know?'*

"Thimerosal was tested only once, by Eli Lilly on the 22 adult patients suffering from meningitis. There was no chance for follow-up to observe long-term effects, as all the patients in this 'study' died. Even if follow-up had been possible, damage to the developing brains of very young children would have remained unknown. Eli Lilly said it was safe and the medical community accepted it. After the creation of the FDA, its use was simply continued. The federal government has never tested the type of mercury in vaccines for toxicity. This is an unconscionable oversight failure at best, at worse it is an example of how we have left **consensus** reality to be created by the liar's junk scientists employ."

Kenneth P. Stoller, MD. "My Open Letter to the American Academy of Pediatrics":

You can avoid having your child vaccinated by claiming your religious freedom to do so. It is still a Constitutional right for every citizen. The pharmaceutical companies along with their partners in crime the CDC are doing all they can to take ANY right of refusal away for yourself or your child. They continue to bribe and pressure politicians to enact laws that will force you and your family to be vaccinated.

This is what "modern medicine" has to offer to you and your infant when giving birth under their rituals and in their hospitals. If you want to read more about how to sidestep this there are many sources and I will list them at the end of this chapter. I will leave you with an excerpt from July 27th, 2013 from Whiteout press:

Courts quietly confirm MMR Vaccine causes Autism by Mark Wachtler

July 27, 2013. Austin. (ONN) After decades of passionate debate, parents probably missed the repeated admissions by drug companies and governments alike that vaccines do in fact cause autism. For concerned parents seeking the truth, it's worth remembering that the exact same people who own the world's drug companies also own America's news outlets. Finding propaganda-free information has been difficult, until now.

—Dr. Andrew Wakefield

At the center of the fifteen-year controversy is Dr. Andrew Wakefield of Austin, Texas. It was Dr. Wakefield that first publicized the link between stomach disorders and autism, and taking the findings one step further, the link between stomach disorders, autism, and the Measles Mumps Rubella (MMR) vaccine. For that discovery way back in 1996, and a subsequent research paper published by the doctor in 1998, Andrew Wakefield has found himself the victim of a world-wide smear campaign by drug corporations, governments, and media companies. And while Dr. Wakefield has been persecuted and prosecuted to the extent of being unable to legally practice medicine because of his discovery, he has instead become a best-selling author, the founder of the Strategic Autism Initiative, and the Director of the Autism Media Channel.

But in recent months, courts, governments and vaccine manufacturers have quietly conceded the fact that the Measles Mumps Rubella (MMR) vaccine most likely does cause autism and stomach diseases. Pharmaceutical companies have even gone so far as to pay out massive monetary awards, totaling in the millions, to the victims in an attempt to compensate them for damages and to buy their silence.

Landmark rulings

In December 2012, two landmark decisions were announced that confirmed Dr. Wakefield's original concern that there is a link between the MMR vaccine, autism and stomach disorders.

> The important thing to say is that back in 1996–1997 I was made aware of children developing autism, regressive autism, following exposure in many cases to the measles mumps rubella vaccine. Such was my concern about the safety of that vaccine that I went back and reviewed every safety study, every pre-licensing study of the MMR vaccine and other measles-containing vaccines before they were put into children and after. And I was appalled with the quality of

that science. It really was totally below par and that has been reiterated by other authoritative sources since.

All I could do as a parent was to say, "what would I do for my child?" That was the only honest answer I could give. My position on that has not changed. So, what happened subsequently? At that time the single measles vaccines were available freely on the National Health Service. Otherwise, I would not have suggested that option. So parents, if they were legitimately concerned about the safety of MMR could go and get the single vaccines. Six months later, the British government unilaterally withdrew the importation license for the single vaccines, therefore depriving parents of having these on the NHS; depriving parents who had legitimate concerns about the safety of MMR from a choice; denying them the opportunity to protect their children in the way that they saw fit.

And I was astonished by this and I said to Dr. Elizabeth Miller of the Health Protection Agency, "why would you do this if your principal concern is to protect children from serious infectious disease? Why would you remove an option from parents who are legitimately concerned about the safety of MMR?" And her answer was extraordinary. She said to me, "if we allow parents the option of single vaccines, it would destroy our MMR program." In other words, her principal concern seemed to be full protection of the MMR program and not protection of children.

Dr. Wakefield himself reiterates the final conclusion of the courts in various countries, but censored by the world's media outlets saying:

"Now this question has been answered not by me, but by the courts, by the vaccine courts in Italy and in the United States of America where it appears that many children over the last thirty years have been awarded millions of dollars for the fact that they have been brain-damaged by MMR vaccine and other vaccines and that brain damage has led to autism. That is a fact."

We need more doctors, health officials and politicians like Dr. Andrew Wakefield who is a friend to the People and an enemy of corruption, greed and those that will endanger you and your families life for a big payday. There are decent people who work at CDC, NIH and other government agencies and a few decent, honest politicians but the fact is that corruption is prevalent and flagrant throughout the pharmaceutical and political world. Most of the populace will never hear about this because the mainstream media is just as corrupt as they are.

According to several studies from Microbe Inotech Laboratories Inc, St Louis Missouri, Monsanto's poison-ous weed killer called Roundup (glyphosate) has been found in numerous vaccines.

Dr. Toni Bark, founder and medical director of the Center for Disease Prevention and Reversal and co-producer of the movie BOUGHT, had this to say after reviewing the test results:

"I am deeply concerned about injecting glypho-sate, a known pesticide, directly into children. Neither Roundup nor glyphosate has been tested for safety as an injectable. Injection is a very different route of entry than the oral route. Injected toxins, even in minute doses can have profound effects on the organs and the different systems of the body. In addition, injecting a chemical along with an adjuvant or live virus, can induce severe allergic reactions to that substance as vaccines induce the immune system to create antibodies to whatever is included in the vaccine. Since glyphosate is heavily used in corn, soy, wheat, cotton and other commodities, we can expect to see more severe food allergies in the vaccine recipients. In addition, chemicals in ultra-low doses can have powerful effects on physiology behaving almost as hormones, stimulating or suppressing physiological receptors."

"This calls for independent scientists, without financial ties to Monsanto, to investigate these findings, and if verified, immediate regulatory and legislative action," said Robert F. Kennedy, Jr., co-founder of The Mercury Project. *"Lawyers litigating against Monsanto should be looking into the company's awareness of this contamination and its effect on children. The public needs to be ready for Monsanto and vaccine manufacturer backlash by their PR machines on this potentially grave information."*

The fact is Big Pharma WANTS your child sick and dependent on their drugs as quickly as possible. The early vaccination protocol can assure them and their investors that no history of health is evident if the child is immediately poisoned by their vaccines. This is a scheme that protects them from future lawsuits and ensures big profits.

Given all this information on birthing your child, is it any wonder that so many children are shut down, sick, become "autistic," or simply die in childbirth? This bizarre onslaught of medical dysfunction and interference needs to be avoided to keep you and your baby safe. If you think this is an exaggeration about the damaging effects of doctors, hospitals and drug companies on childbirth maybe this will change your mind.

From Michelle Castillo at CBS News (5/7/13), "About 11,300 newborns die within 24 hours of their birth in the U.S. each year, 50 percent more first-day deaths than all other industrialized countries combined."

She goes on to say *"Worldwide, the report found that 800 women die each day during pregnancy or childbirth, and 8,000 newborns die during the first month of life. Newborn deaths make up 43 percent of all deaths for children under five. Sixty percent of infant deaths occur during the first month of life."*

The top five countries to be a mom were Finland, Sweden, Norway, Iceland and the Netherlands. The bottom five were Niger, Mali, Sierra Leone, Somalia and the Democratic Republic of the Congo.

Because of their high infant mortality rates, the U.S. only ranked number 30 this year on the report, down five spots from the 2012 report. Save the Children CEO Carolyn Miles told CBSNews.com she was shocked to find that out that the U.S. ranked so low.

According to worldstatinfo.com, 2015, the US is 50th in the world for infant mortality rates. According to the

14th annual State of the World's Mothers report calculated by Save The Children, the United States is 51st. On the CIA's list, the US ranks 44th in infant mortality.

If that is not shocking enough for you to think that the present medical model for childbirth is a failure I don't know what would be. The fact is, as Dr. Robert Mendelsohn said: "Whenever you are in a hospital you are in mortal danger." That goes for your baby as well.

My suggestion is to get yourself extremely healthy, educate yourself about natural, drug-free childbirth. If you feel like a home birth is too scary then you could go to a hospital birthing center, where it feels less like a hospital and you have a chance to get your baby out with little or no harm done. Exercise and demand your religious freedom to prevent poisons from entering your child bloodstream. Interview a bunch of midwives and Doulas' to assist you. Speak to and listen to as many mothers who have given birth naturally, drug free and at home.

Understand that most doctors and pharmaceutical companies will do their very best and spend big money to scare you into doing things that you don't want to do. Fear and deception is their weapon, Knowledge is yours. Your best protection is Knowledge of the birth process. A complete understanding of all the risks involved and all the remedies to those risks. As mentioned before, bringing a child into the world is a Huge responsibility and by gaining an Understanding of the process you will KNOW for yourself what the right choices are. One of the best books I know on this topic is Ina May's *Guide to Childbirth*. It is a no-nonsense comprehensive book that helps you to get a true understanding of what childbirth was meant to look like. Make a study of this book (and a couple of others mentioned at the end of this chapter) It will save you and your baby from a lot of dangerous and unnecessary situations and "treatments."

As a parent/guardian, you have the responsibility to ensure that your child is protected from the absurd and dangerous madness imposed by "modern medicine." Ideally, they should be born at home in a quiet dimly lit room with one or two people around speaking in soft tones and communicating with themselves and others with consciousness. A relaxed, prepared, courageous and celebratory tone should be set by the mother and those surrounding her. There is no need to be afraid if you are truly educated, prepared and have a birthing expert with you. The people present should be the Father/and or coach and the birth assistant (midwife and/or Doula). It helps to have a couple of other capable family members or close friends who are supportive and in goodwill towards you nearby or in other parts of the house. If a home birth really scares you can always ask a friend or relative to sit outside your house while in labor to drive you to a hospital if needed.

Breastfeeding

Breastfeeding is a vitally important stage in the child's development. Not just physically and mentally but emotionally as well. Who can argue that it is one of the most natural acts known to humanity? Those who argue are the ones who are profiting from the sale of "formula," and/or have been brainwashed and mis-educated. Breastfeeding has shown to help the Mother physically recover faster and end any bleeding or swelling that might occur after birth.

Human breast milk varies from one mother to the next. It is precisely designed by nature for your specific baby. In fact, studies show that the same mother will have different amounts of sugar, fat, and protein according to what child they are birthing. The colostrum, the original milk produced by the mother lines your baby's intestinal wall and can prevent many childhood digestive problems and allergies. Every child has its own specific needs and requirements to be healthy and your body knows exactly what ingredients these are and will produce them. Providing cooked, drugged and steroid-laced milk from a cow (re-read the chapter on dairy products) or a denatured indigestible powdered formula from a box is sure to create Serious deficiencies and health problems for your baby, including ear infections, constipation, gas, stomach pain, headaches, excess mucus skin rashes and more. There are thousands of useful components in Human breast milk that science can identify and most likely thousands more that they haven't yet identified. None of them can be reproduced in a lab or by a candy company.

Never give your child "baby formula." No matter what the manufacturer's claims are or what your doctor tells you. They are filled with ingredients that simply do not belong in a human body let alone an infant's.

One large study by the National Institute of Environmental Health Sciences showed that children who are breastfed have a 20 percent lower risk of dying between the ages of 28 days and 1 year than children who weren't breastfed, with longer breastfeeding associated with lower risk.

Scientists think that immune factors such as secretory IgA (only available in breast milk) help prevent allergic reactions to food by providing a layer of protection to a baby's intestinal tract. Without this protection, inflammation can develop and the wall of the intestine can become porous or "leaky." This allows undigested proteins to cross the gut where they can cause an allergic reaction and other health problems. Babies who are fed formula rather than breast milk don't get this layer of protection, so they're more vulnerable to inflammation, intestinal sensitivities, allergies, and other illnesses.

Nature knows better than the food corporations . . . . Much better.

Breastfeeding is not a step you can "skip" without grave consequences to your child and deleterious effects to yourself. There has been a lot of evidence and study results that show that mothers who breastfeed their infants have a much lower risk of postpartum depression. The skin to skin contact with your baby provides a chemical exchange between Mother and child that is being scientifically proven to aid both child and mother. There is increasing evidence that skin to skin contact between mother and child has tremendous benefits to both mother and child. Babies who have consistent contact with their mother tend to cry less stabilize their breathing easier, stabilize their heart rates better and stabilize their blood glucose.

Some women have difficulty getting the child to latch on to their breasts and/or find it painful at first.

This is only because of lack of knowledge. There are women who teach this to first-time mothers. They are called lactation coaches and it would be a great idea to ask your doula, midwife or birth assistant about this well before your baby is born if you can get help on the birthday of your child.

According to Linda Palmer a Chiropractor and author of another fine book on pregnancy and childbirth called *Baby Matters*, says

> "Prolactin is released in all healthy people during sleep, helping to maintain reproductive organs and immune function. In the mother, prolactin is released in response to suckling, promoting milk production as well as maternal behaviors. Prolactin relaxes mother, and in the early months, creates a bit of fatigue during a nursing session so she has no strong desire to hop up and do other thing Prolactin promotes caregiving behaviors and, over time, directs brain reorganization to favor these behaviors. Father's prolactin levels begin to elevate during mother's pregnancy, but most of the rise in the male occurs after many days of cohabitation with the infant."

> "Persistent regular body contact and other nurturing acts by parents produce a constant, elevated level of oxytocin in the infant, which in turn provides a valuable reduction in the infant's stress-hormone responses. Multiple psychology studies have demonstrated that, depending on

the practices of the parents, the resulting high or low level of oxytocin will control the permanent organization of the stress-handling portion of the baby's brain—promoting lasting "securely attached" or "insecure" characteristics in the adolescent and adult. Such insecure characteristics include antisocial behavior, aggression, difficulty forming lasting bonds with a mate, mental illness, and poor handling of stress. When an infant does not receive regular oxytocin-producing responsive care, the resultant stress responses cause elevated levels of the stress hormone cortisol. Chronic cortisol elevations in infants and the hormonal and functional adjustments that go along with it are shown in biochemical studies to be associated with permanent brain changes that lead to elevated responses to stress throughout life, such as higher blood pressure and heart rate. Mothers can also benefit from the stress-reducing effects of oxytocin-women who breastfeed produce significantly less stress hormone than those who bottle-feed."

How to avoid morning sickness

The reason "morning sickness" is so common is simple. When your body is pregnant it will do everything it can to keep the baby's environment clean. When eating the Standard American Diet or anything close to it your body is being continually poisoned at an average of 50 times per day. Because your body is in "pregnancy mode" it will be more acutely compelled to rid your body of poisons to protect the baby. While you are sleeping your body will be working to purge itself, release poisons into the bloodstream and when you awake the body will push the poisons out. Vomiting is the quickest way for your body to do that. If you wish to avoid morning sickness stop eating a poisoned diet. "Morning sickness" does not exist for those that eat according to their biology, organic, raw fruits, vegetables, seeds, and nuts.

General care of the child

Sleeping

A newborn infant will sleep a large part of the day, usually about 16–18 hrs. Sleep patterns can vary and as the child gets older he/ she may sleep less and change the pattern. Make sure to change your baby's diaper as soon as possible in order to avoid diaper rash, which can be extremely irritating and painful. You may have to do this about 8 to 10 times per day. Make sure the baby is not too cold or too hot. Try sleeping when the baby does and you will feel more rested.

Sign Language

A lot of parents get extremely frustrated when their child cries for extended periods of time. The crying is a request.

You must figure out what that request is. Crying is the only way an infant can communicate their needs. It is very inefficient, as the parent cannot tell what the baby needs. That is, unless you teach the child sign language. Take the time to learn 15 or 20 signs and teach them to your baby. A child as young as 5 or 6 months can begin to learn simple signs and by age 1 you can really communicate well with each other. Besides being very useful it is very amusing and satisfying as well. Your child's communication skills will already be somewhat developed by the time they use words.

The sign for hungry and thirsty is very simple. Every time you feed the child or give them something to drink simply say out loud "drink" or "eat" while repeating the appropriate sign, two or three times so they can see it. Also, take their little hand and direct it to make the sign for themselves right before they get to drink/eat and as they are drinking or eating. After repeating this regularly they will begin to ask through their sign language for what they want. It is quite remarkable. You have to be consistent and you must be patient and cheerful while teaching them.

Here is a list of what infants cry for: Breast milk, food, diaper change, sleep, too hot, too cold, too much light, too much darkness, wants to be held, wants to sleep, wants to be put down on the ground, stuck in child seat or stroller and/or wants to get out (there is a sign for "later" and in a "few minutes") a desire to be read to, played with, or have a certain toy.

Once the baby knows the sign for yes or no and for the above needs and wants you will virtually wipe out all crying for long periods of time. This will create a lot more harmony and peace for all involved and more sleep. It is quite magical and extremely satisfying to have the ability to clearly communicate with your baby before the child can speak.

Make sure to learn the sign for "more," "I have had enough" and "Thank you" and "I Love You."

If your baby is crying, try to figure out what can be done to help. A change of diapers, something to eat or drink, or soothing some physical discomfort. After you have done that it may be that the child wants the mother but she is not available. It could be that the child has been frightened by a loud noise or startled by something it has seen. Maybe the clothes are too hot or too tight. Be patient.

If you have tried everything and the baby is still crying try this: Hold the child firmly but allow it space to move its arms and head. The child may twist and convulse while in the throes of a tantrum. Begin to pat the child firmly on the back with a quick rhythm Imagine your beat is matching the baby's heart rate keep it going for a minute or so till you have a certain rhythmic connection with the child. Then begin to slow it down imperceptibly at first, then slower and slower. Slow it down to about 1 beat per second. After a few minutes, your child will be much calmer and may even fall asleep. I know there is a proposed method where "experts" are advising to ignore the crying child and let it "self-soothe." That is ignorant, cruel, absurd and only makes the child feel abandoned. There will be plenty of time to teach your child how to soothe themselves when they get older. If your child is less than seven years old always pay attention and do all you can to comfort the child. You must do your best to sleep when the baby sleeps. At least for the first 6 or 7 months. Eventually, your baby will get a sleep rhythm naturally.

Babies and infants will often grab at your face and/ or hit. Do not get upset or impatient. They mean no harm but simply want to explore the surface and texture of your face. Gently and continually redirect their hands to your shoulder, you can let them hit you there where it will be much less painful and tolerable. You can also show them how to touch your face gently by taking their little hands and putting them on your face in a gentle sooth- ing manner. If you repeat the word "gentle" while doing this eventually your child will understand. Some older toddlers will also hit when frustrated. You must NOT hit them back but teach them that hitting is simply not allowed and tell them that they must use their words to express themselves.

I do not recommend pacifiers. Besides eating, babies use their mouths mostly to explore and putting a piece of plastic in your child's mouth is not a good idea.

Water

Tap water is filled with poisons. Besides Chlorine and Fluoride, (both deadly chemicals) there is lead, mercury, arsenic etc.

Make sure you have a solid water filter and/or access to clean water, NEVER drink tap water especially while pregnant or leading up to your pregnancy.

As mentioned before in this book there are basic elements required for life and good health. A loving atten- tive, responsible parent/guardian(s), fresh air, sunshine, clean water and nutritious food are essential components.

The water supply in this country has been poisoned. Get a water purifier for your home that eliminates chlorine, lead, and fluoride, three highly toxic poisons that cause disease. Get water purifiers for your shower heads as well so you are not showering with chlorine. You can buy a charcoal-filled bath filter that comes in a plastic ball that you can swirl around the bathtub to eliminate chlorine in the bath water. If you are unable or unwilling to be 100% raw during your pregnancy then insist on at least %70 raw diet with no animal products and make a real effort to ingest no poisons including tap water.

Sun

It is a good idea to allow your newborn some time in the mild morning sun (Sunrise to 10 am) for about 5 to 10 minutes a day. Preferably naked on the grass (as long as the grass has not been sprayed with pesticides.) If that is not possible the evening sun (4 pm to sunset) will do as well. Make sure it is no more than 10 minutes. Avoid any lengthy exposure in the midday sun with infants and small children.

Saying that the "Sun causes cancer" is the same thing as saying that "water causes drowning." If you keep your head under water too long you will drown. If you overexpose yourself too long and too often to the Sun over the years you will damage your skin. Yet both Water and Sunshine are essential for good health. All adults should spend at least 20 minutes a day in the sun.

Sunscreen

Most sunscreens are toxic. Avoid them. When your child is in the sun skin pores are opened and these toxins are absorbed by the body. There is no need for sunscreen. Use common sense and keep your child out of the sun for extended periods of time. Never allow your child to get sunburned. It is painful and damaging to the skin. Teach them how to tell when the sun is burning them. Obviously, the lighter the skin your child has the more careful you must be. As your child begins to tan the skin will become less sensitive and the child can stay out longer. Overexposure can be as bad as underexposure.

If your child insists on being in the midday sun too long there are solutions. There are many natural brands of sunscreen that are not toxic. Obviously covering the skin with clothing that will prevent sunburn in most cases is a good solution. If it is really hot outside you can soak their shirt and pants in water then put them back on to stay cool and protected from sunburn.

Cosmetics

Most commercial cosmetics, like most pharmaceutical drugs, are petroleum-based products. They are extremely toxic. Lipsticks, foundation, perfume etc. are absorbed into the bloodstream through the skin. Cosmetics are the cause of many health problems and you should do your best to use only the most natural, non-petroleum based products. Wearing these cosmetics while with your baby can harm their health. This goes for soaps and shampoos as well. Buy only petroleum free, alcohol-free, animal product-free items.

Teeth

Teething pain is a natural occurrence and can start as early as 5 or 6 months. In some babies, it is more painful than others. Some children will develop a slight fever while teething, which is normal. No need to panic. The best thing you can do is make sure the rest of their body is comfortable and not too hot. A cool rag on the head can help. A frozen teething ring can be useful as well (you can take strips of cloth towels and wet them then put them in the freezer in a ring or a pretzel-like shape for them to chew on once it is frozen). You can also just take a face rag or small towel and wet the corner and put it in the freezer for them to chew on. If the baby is still in pain you can use some Arnica gel on the gums. You will be able to find this at your local health food store. You can also try clove oil, you may need to dilute it and apply a little bit on the gums where the teeth are coming in as it will help to numb the area.

Some young children will develop small cavities in their teeth. This is NOT a problem unless it becomes painful. If your child is abiding by a natural raw or mostly raw diet the teeth will not be painful or sensitive. These are baby teeth and they will eventually fall out, dental procedures are not necessary. Teeth are made more sensitive by eating cooked, denatured, processed foods. Avoid all acid producing foods pasteurized juices, soda, refined sugar, processed food etc.

Contact with the earth

It is a health-giving natural act to have your child in direct contact with the grass and the soil. Walking (or crawling) barefoot is a scientifically-researched practice with a number of remarkable health advantages, such as increasing antioxidants, reducing inflammation, and improved sleep. Studies are showing that the health benefits come from the relationship between our bodies and the electrons in the earth. The planet has its own natural charge, and human beings are healthier when we're in direct contact with it instead of wearing shoes all the time.

A review published in the Journal of Environmental and Public Health looked at a number of studies that highlight how drawing electrons from the earth improves health.

Another study found that being in direct contact with Earth changed the electrical activity in the brain, as measured by electroencephalograms. Still, other research found that being in direct contact with the earth moderated heart rate variability, improved glucose regulation, reduced stress and boosted immunity.

Besides these findings, it just makes sense that human beings were meant to keep their bodies in contact with the earth. So you and your baby should be barefoot in the grass, or on the beach on a daily basis.

Cleaning Products

Most commercial cleaning products from dish soap, laundry detergent, and household cleaning products are poisonous. They can irritate your skin and eyes, pollute our water supply and are disastrous to our ecology. Avoid them. Buy ONLY nontoxic cleaners. Cleaning your house with hazardous materials is NOT really useful and antithetical to the purpose of cleaning. There are many house hold cleaners on the market that are safe and non-toxic. Also, Vinegar is extremely effective at cleaning windows, bathtubs toilets and getting rid of mold. Try putting vinegar in a spray bottle and see how well it cleans. Take 30 minutes to educate yourself on safe household cleaners. Refuse to buy ANY product that will harm the environment.

Clothing

You should do your best to keep nothing but organic cotton clothes on your child. Avoid polyester and other fake materials, especially those that touch the skin. They are irritants to the child's skin. If your child is wearing a belt (or pants with a waistband) make sure it is not too tight as that can cause digestive problems. Obviously, you want to make sure your baby is warm enough. At the same time, it is important for the child to be naked as much as possible, especially during the warmer months. I know that diapers are necessary for our civilized world but they are extremely unnatural. Keeping the child with

urine and feces pressed against its skin is bound to produce skin irritation and pain and discomfort. Obviously
change your baby as quickly as you can and allow your
child to be naked as much as possible as long as it is warm
enough.

If your child does have diaper rash that means that
you are not changing the baby quickly enough. There
are many natural ointments and soothing gels for this.
Choose the one with the least additives and toxin free.
There are some products on the market that are safe. Also,
make sure your baby knows the sign for diaper change.

Toilet training

If you are lucky enough to have a backyard and can keep
the child safe it would be best to do so without diapers.
If you have taught your baby sign language the child can
tell you when he/she has to go to the bathroom. Getting
a small toilet (or a child's seat for your home toilet) is a
good way to train them. If you give praise and rewards
to your child for going in the toilet he/she will be happy
to do it every time. Something as simple as a paper with
gold stars every time they use the toilet instead of diapers
will work along with a lot of praise and before you know
it your child be able to go without diapers. It is important
to explain to them how a toilet works and that is completely safe and there is no way they can be flushed away.
Many small children have this fear of the toilet and the
bathtub. It is your job to explain it in a fun understand-
able way that alleviates their fears.

It is also important to realize that your child up until the age of 7 or 8 could have accidents. It is very important not to punish or shame them. Treat them with love and understanding. Do not make a big deal out of it. Take them aside and privately clean them up and ask them what happened and why is it they didn't get to the toilet on time. Explain to them that they are not in trouble and that this happens to all children at some time or another. Tell them it even happens to adults. Listen closely to their answer and consider what they are telling you. Ask them if you can help. Ask them what they could do differently next time so that they can get to the bathroom on time. Give them extra hugs and reassurance.

Baby food

Your baby can breastfeed for a long time. The amount of time is often influenced by cultural norms but there are children that will breastfeed until the age of 5 or 6. Some children will decide to stop on their own and sometimes mothers and their children can make a mutual agreement to wean.

The American Academy of Pediatrics supports mothers who want to nurse as long as necessary. "It's completely appropriate that a mother should avail herself to her infant or toddler," said Dr. Lori Winter, of the American Academy of Pediatrics. "That's in no way damaging to the child." The American Academy of Pediatrics recommends nursing up to one year and as long as mutually desired by the mother and the child.

Studies even have shown extended nursing has great health benefits for the child.

"They don't become as obese as children who are not being breastfed," Winter said. "They have protection against ear infections, diarrhea." Mothers too can benefit from the process. "A mother can reduce her chances of premenopausal breast cancer if she breast-feeds for at least two years," Winter added.

It is important that you do what the child wants in terms of deciding when to stop. By ending breastfeeding too soon it can cause serious stress for an infant or small child. If you decide to stop on your own without your child's consent then I would suggest a lot of extra attention and physical contact. You can include a bottle or sippy cup with coconut water or fresh juices while holding your child. Fresh Carrot juice is a good one to start with. You can begin to mix and match by adding apple juice, spinach, celery, pineapple etc. ONLY organic and fresh NOT pasteurized!

Unfortunately, most baby foods are cooked and nutritionally unsound. Many are filled with sugar and salt and highly processed ingredients. Avoid them. Your baby will begin to reach for food when he/she is ready to eat. All babies will differ as to what time they will start wanting solid foods.

For babies with no teeth or just a couple of teeth, you have to be careful. Do not feed the infant any food that requires chewing. Mashed-up bananas are very easy for a baby to eat and taste delicious. You can use a fork to do this. You can do the same with berries, apples (blender, food processor) and avocados. Please make sure the fruit is organic and ripe. You can tell a ripe banana by the absence of green any skin (should be all yellow) and the brown spots that will begin to appear on the skin. An avocado is ripe when firm with a little softness to it, akin to a stick of refrigerated butter. Eating unripe fruit is very disruptive to the digestive tract, the fruit will stay acid in the digestive system and cause problems and pain. Overripe fruit or fermenting fruit will also cause problems. It is overripe when the fruit smells like alcohol and becomes too soft. Give your baby only foods at room temperature. Avoid ALL pasteurized juices. They are acidic and can damage the teeth and stomach lining.

You can make all kinds of fresh juices and your baby will love them (and you too!) Start off with plain freshly squeezed orange, apple or carrot juice. You can begin to add other fruits and vegetables and see what the child prefers. Carrot apple is a delicious combination as is carrot spinach but the combinations are endless. I would suggest at first only a plain fruit or vegetable juice to see how the child responds. Pure apple juice or carrot juice is a great start.

If you can get fresh coconuts, buy a cleaver and learn how to open them. The water inside is incredibly nutritious as is the coconut flesh. You can blend the two to make your child a delicious shake. You can add a banana and even some raw almond butter for a meal-like coconut "milkshake." There is also a brand of coconut water called Harmless Harvest, and now a few others, that are not cooked, organic and very delicious and nutritious.

Some thoughts on parenting

Your baby, from conception to the age of 7 is VERY impressionable. Everything seen, heard and felt can make an imprint like a photographic plate and will contribute to how the child forms into an adult. Yes, even in the womb.

When pregnant, it is important for both parents to talk and/or sing to the child on a daily basis. As soon as you know you are pregnant you can begin talking to the child in soothing tones about how happy you are that he/she is here and what a wonderful life awaits them. Playing soothing music from Bach, Beethoven, Mozart, Mendelssohn, Vivaldi is highly recommended. Of course, there are many other composers and types of music that is soothing. In my opinion, these composers are the finest and their music has an extremely comforting effect.

When your child is 6 or 7 months in utero you can even play games with them by very gently pushing or gently tapping on them while in the womb. It helps to do it in rhythm to a song that you are singing or a song that is playing so you can both hear. You will notice after the 8th month that the child will often push back, sometimes in rhythm. Sing to the child in utero. You should probably do that in private so you are not thought to be nuts. By doing these activities you already have created a playful, welcoming bond with your baby before it is born.

Once the child is born he /she will already be around familiar sounds and people it has known for 9 months. This will be very comforting and a huge help to the infant. Continue with the music and the singing.

Time is much different for children. Try to remember when you were a child of 6 or 7 how long a summer day seemed to last. Children are more awake and conscious than most adults. Always keep this in mind when dealing with your child. If you are unhappy, short or impatient with your child for 5 minutes it may seem like nothing to you but an eternity for them.

The opposite is true as well. When you are fully engaged with your child and you are both enjoying yourselves it will be a great gift and a huge boon to your child that will seem endless in time.

Discipline

Discipline comes from the word disciple. A person who learns from another. You are responsible for preparing your child for their adult life and to teach them how to control themselves and take care of themselves. That means YOU must control yourself. You will get plenty of opportunities every day to do so once your child is born. Please practice patience, consideration, and selflessness. You most likely have had little or no effective training in teaching a child, so you are going to have to study and retrain yourself to raise the child without doing any damage.

NEVER hit your child. It creates immediate distrust and confusion and is shocking, demoralizing and humiliating and a sure way to crush your child's self-esteem which can and will cause a plethora of physical and emotional problems in the future. Most violent criminals have histories of being beaten by their parents. There is NEVER A "GOOD REASON" TO HIT YOUR CHILD. It doesn't matter what your parents did, or what you think is right. YOU must learn patience and tolerance if you wish to be a decent parent and raise a child who will help humanity. If you must discipline your child there are countless ways to do it without hitting and demeaning them. Time outs work beautifully.

The best way to change your child's behavior is by being very clear (what is expected and why) and by repeating exactly what you desire over and over again and have them do that very thing. Applaud and encourage them when they behave and do what is asked of them. Instead of repeating "no, no" or "don't do that," continually tell them and show them what you want them to do. Be patient. It takes time for a child to develop good habits. You will be rewarded for your patience and your child will be grateful.

Yelling at your child can be extremely damaging and destructive. It is a form of violence. Never do it unless the child is in grave danger. Never tease your child, for ANY reason. Never call your child derogatory names. NEVER. If you do, apologize immediately. Remember that being a Mother or Father you are Gods to the infant or child. You have the ability to give your baby/child beautiful loving impressions that will last their entire lives and continue to enrich them and all they come in contact with, by being patient, playful, intelligent, loving and considerate to all their needs. You will be required to be stern and serious with your child from time to time. You must learn how to get their attention with a facial expression and serious tone of voice.

If you make the effort to see the world new and see the world through their eyes you will not only be less frustrated and angry, you too will become more alive, younger and more playful.

By raising your child in a loving thoughtful manner you also get to share and have experiences that you may have never had as a child. It can be very comforting to give to your child what you never received and very therapeutic for you as well.

Infants and small children are very impressionable. As a parent, it is your duty to make sure that your child is exposed to only the finest impressions. The finest people (in their finest moods), the finest relationships, the finest music, the finest fairy tales and stories, the finest food, the finest language (do not curse or use foul language in front of your children) and the finest love and care you can give them. By making these consistent efforts you will be amazed at the abilities and development of your child. Of course, you are not going to be able to do it all the time. Just do your best and remember that your efforts now will be greatly rewarded in the future.

If you are upset and angry put your child down and /or leave the room until you can control yourself. NEVER fight with your spouse in front of your infant or toddler or any child. NEVER. It is an unbearable sight for a little one to endure the sight and sounds of his/her parents fighting. It is extremely damaging to their psyche and leaves a devastating impression that can never be erased. If you must fight and argue do it outside the sight and sound of your child. Learn to whisper fight in other rooms. You and your husband/wife can make a pact to put the child's well being first and your own selves second. This is a VERY important part of being a loving and effective parent.

Children below the age of seven should never be directly exposed to your personal adult problems. They are children and have many problems of their own. Burdening a child with your adult problems is a form of mental abuse as most children do not have the capacity to understand or think clearly about their mother and father's difficulties especially when there are conflicts between the parents. Do not be emotionally dependent on your child. Remember you are the parent and they need you to be the adult. Keep your adult problems for adults. Also, remember you are the Parent and Guardian of the child, not a friend. Parenthood and Friendship are DIFFERENT. You must always play your role as a Parent. Your child may often times disagree with you and be angry with you for imposing discipline and that is completely normal. They may claim to "hate" you for it in the moment but will be grateful that they have boundaries set and know that you are doing what is in their best interest. You must learn to bear these situations where your child dislikes you. Please watch "Mr. Rogers Talks With Parents About Discipline" on YouTube.

Do NOT let your children be programmed by television. Do NOT let your children sit in front of the TV or a computer screen to entertain themselves or give you "a break." Remember that children are extremely impressionable. Remember it is called TELEVISION PROGRAMMING for a reason. Do you want programmed children? I recommend NO TV. It would be wise to bring your child up without any television. Commercial television will rot your child's mind.

Get them in the habit of reading at a very early age. The best way to do this is to read to them for at least one or two hours a day. End the day with a bedtime story. I highly recommend Aesops Fables, Grimm's Fairy Tales (unedited), Little Women (Alcott), Little House on the Prairie (Laura Wilder), Charles Dickens, Mark Twain, Hans Christian Anderson, The Wizard Of Oz and Herman Hesse's Fairy Tales. Not only are these stories and authors incredibly entertaining there is a moral code and standard that run through all of them.

The same goes for video games, computer screens, phones, and tablets. DO NOT allow children to use electronics as a source of activity. Reading, music, art, board games and puzzles are activities that will develop your child's mind. INSIST that your child does some kind of physical activity on a daily basis. Whether it's playing tag, riding bicycles, skipping rope, roller-blading, skateboarding or just playing at the playground. Physical activity is necessary for your child's well being. They should be in motion a minimum of 1 hour per day.

IF you MUST have your children watch TV allow them to watch commercial free. I would highly suggest Mister Rogers Neighborhood. The shows are intelligent, kind-hearted, musical, uplifting and very educational as well as geared for a child's mind. Also, your child will not be bombarded with special effects, overstimulation, constant viewing cuts, mind control, poor behavior or anything offensive.

There are other books and TV shows recommended at the end of this chapter.

Reading

Teaching your child to read is very simple, if you have some patience. It is also incredibly fun as every day they will improve. You can start to teach them as young as two years of age. Show them the alphabet. Start by singing the alphabet song together. Then point to a letter and repeat the sound/s it makes. Do it repeatedly, until they can do it themselves. Then (for instance) show them the letters "at." Repeat the sound these letters make a few times, then have them do it. Congratulate them when they get it right. Then put a c in front of that word. Point to the three letters and say the word "cat" aloud 3 or 4 times. Ask them to do it. Praise them a lot when they get it right.

The bigger your response the more willing they will be to get the next one right. . . . Being a little over the top here just adds to the enjoyment. Start with a normal response, "good job!" then increase your joy each time they get it right. Try falling off the couch every once in awhile if they get it right 3X in a row . . . Smack yourself in the head (open hand recommended) and beat your child with pillows when they get it right too often (as long as your child likes that sort of pillow beating, most kids do. Obviously take it easy on them) all the while yelling "how can you be so smart." You get the idea . . . make it fun, an event that brings laughter joy and the unexpected . . . When they get it wrong simply say in an encouraging tone "let's try again." Or you can make an absurdly loud buzzer sound and yell "Buzzer of wrongness!" (don't make that too fun . . . could lead to problems).

Keep repeating what the correct pronunciation is. Then put a "b" in front of "at" and repeat the word 3 or 4 times. Have them say the word. Keep changing the first letter from c to s to b to r to f to h to m and back to c. Praising your child each time they get it right as your praise will inspire them to keep going. Then change the root from "at" to "ig" . . . You get the idea. Pretty soon they will be so eager to learn more and if you make it fun they will want to read all day. You can have a scoreboard and keep score of how many words/pages they get right. Also you can give little prizes if they get a certain amount right. By the time they are 2 or 2½ they will be able to read simple books. The feeling of pride alone will give your child such joy as well as open up an entire new world for them. Remember to have fun and laugh a lot. NO negativity. ONLY positive reinforcement. Try to make it fun for both of you. Some kids might not be responsive at first. Don't be impatient, laugh it off and try something else.

By doing this you will also create more time for yourself as your child will begin to read and entertain themselves by age 3 or 4 . . . without TV or video games. It is likely that they will become avid readers as books provide constant entertainment for their young minds and really exercise their imagination. Make sure you have enough books in the house for them at all times. Join your local library and get your child a library card. You can tell your child "when you are able to read this entire book (*Cat in the Hat*), "you will get your own library card!"

Make a big deal out of any visit to the library. "Today we are going to a building that is FILLED with books and we get to take out any book we want and read it, we even get to take it home!" Find out what kinds of books attract them the most.

Dr. Seuss books are like a carnival to children, as most children love when words rhyme. The *Cat in the Hat* is a perfect start. Read to them the simplest Dr. Seuss books, to begin with. Point to the words as you read them. Then give them a chance to say the word that will rhyme next. Then you can move on to the more difficult ones like Oh *The Places You'll Go* and *The Lorax*.

Most children will catch on very quickly although some may not. Do not be disappointed and try other techniques. Boys and some girls like to keep moving while learning so you can reward them by letting them run to other side of the room let them run in a big circle once they get a word or two or three correct. If after a week or so your child is not catching on, move on to something else or just read to them. Then try again in a week or two. Keep learning fun for both of you.

Music

It is imperative to teach children the basics of music. If you don't have any musical training, get an inexpensive piano or an electronic keyboard and learn with your child. The whole world is made up of vibrating atoms and molecules. There is rhythm to life. Learning music opens up new and useful pathways in the brain. It will teach them math, patience, concentration, and reward for hard work. It is also extremely satisfying to be able to play a song they love. I suggest singing to your child in soothing tones and even making up silly songs about them and your life together. Singing songs is very loving and keeps the child fully engaged. While changing diapers, getting ready for bed, taking a trip to the library, or going for a walk. It is fun to have songs to go along with those activities. Moving the baby's hands and having them clap along is usually a very fun experience for your infant. It can be done easily be sitting with them at the piano, playing scales and simple tunes and singing along. Also teaching a child rhythm is extremely satisfying and appealing. Through music, many lessons can be learned and many parts of the brain that ordinarily would not be accessed become involved.

Also, children love music. Musical education will develop your child's mind like nothing else. Get the soundtrack from The Sound of Music. The music is fun and filled with catchy, easy to learn songs. Learn the words and sing along. Continually play the songs and your child will begin to sing along with you. Sing with them and perhaps dance with them in your arms or when they are old enough hold hands and dance with them around the room. Make it a daily ritual and before you know it they will have their favorite songs and will be learning how to sing and clap along while their brains will be absorbing so much information on rhythm, coordination and the scales of music and the universe.

Chess

Most children love board games. I cannot think of a better board game than chess. At the age of three, you can start teaching your child chess. If done with a sense of fun and reward, "now we get to play chess," your child will love it. If you don't know how to play, learn with them.

The game teaches so many valuable lessons of life such as patience, self-reliance, self-control, how to abide by rules, problem solving, thinking clearly under pressure, anticipation, probability, dealing with unexpected results, recognizing successful and unsuccessful patterns, how to deal with losing, how to deal with winning, holding different ideas in the mind at the same time and sportsmanship. It is a good idea to start every game off with a "good luck" and a firm handshake while making eye contact.

> "Chess is in many ways like life itself. It's all condensed in a playful manner in a game format and it's extremely fascinating because first of all, I'm in control of my own destiny, I'm in charge. You have to be responsible for your actions, you make a move, you had better think ahead about what's going to happen, not after it happens because then it's too late. Chess teaches discipline from a very early age. It teaches you to have a plan and to plan ahead. If you do that, you'll be rewarded; if you break the rules, you will get punished in life and in chess. You need to learn the rules to break the rules."

—Susan Polgar, 4 time World Champion and
founder of the Susan Polgar Foundation.

Art

There are many forms of art from drawing to sculpting
to painting to etching and on and on. Give a child some
crayons and paper and they can be busy for hours. Getting
them exposure to some lessons and they may become
even more interested especially if you do it together. Art
can teach patience, observation, hand-eye coordination,
perspective, appreciation, confidence and so many other
lessons.

Whether it is drawing, sculpting or painting taking
time to be creative and express yourself is always a beneficial habit. Get your kids interested in one of these art
forms and if they express repeated interest, nurture and
encourage their learning and provide what they need to
continue.

People

Be wary of who you allow your baby or young child to
spend time with. Insist that only the most loving people
are allowed to handle and care for the child. Insist that
your home be a cheerful, loving sanctuary where the child
feels safe, calm and cared for. Each parent should take
responsibility for the vibration tone and atmosphere of
the home at all times.

There is a wise precept that says: "Give me the child for the first seven years and I'll show you the man."

Because children are SO impressionable in their first seven years many wise people believed that it did not matter what happened afterward as long as the child received the highest quality love, nurturing, guidance and education in the first seven years.

Manners

Manners are a form of love and respect. Do you want your children to be loving and respectful? Good Manners can be learned by mere repetition but as your child grows older he/she will begin to see the positive effect it has on others and how manners are, in fact, a form of consideration and love. Teach them good manners. You will be happy you did. Of course, that means that you must practice and display good manners at all times. Read Emerson's essay on manners. Teach your sons that they are responsible for protecting women.

Allow your child to take chances.

Having too much can be as damaging as having too little. Being too rich can be as bad, or worse than being poor, eating too much can be more damaging than eating too little and overprotecting your child can be as damaging as neglect. Children who have been "kept safe" are nowhere near as resourceful as those who have had to struggle and take chances. It is wise to keep your child safe but also necessary to allow them to take chances. You have to use your judgment. The greatest experience of our lives usually has occurred while taking chances and or taking risks. Many children today do not get the chance to take risks due to overbearing parents. Learning to be self-sufficient is an invaluable gift you can give to your kids. DO NOT overprotect your kids. Ships are safe in the harbor but that is not what ships are for. There is NO substitute for life experience.

Work

Once your child is past the age of 7 or 8, you may want to begin to treat them as young adults. Start by giving them some adult responsibilities. Whether it is taking out the trash, painting a fence, raking leaves or shoveling snow. Give them tasks to do that are necessary for the functioning of the household. Do it with them a few times so they understand how to do it properly, then have them do it on their own. Praise them when they do it correctly and let them know what they did incorrectly. If they can learn to do simple tasks at an early age their confidence will grow.

Whatever they wish to learn whether it be carpentry, sailing, boxing, mechanics, sculpting or construction try to get them real experience DOING just that. The classroom is NOT real life. Apprenticeship is by FAR the BEST way to learn anything. You do not have to wait until it is offered in a school (which it may never be) or some kind of organized program.

Once your child is 10–12 years old it is important that they find some kind of part-time job. Babysitting, delivery boy, mowing lawns, tutoring, etc. If they want a new bike, guitar, drum set, trampoline. Tell them "You have to earn half of the money for it and I'll pay the other half." Some kids who are hard workers may wish to pay for it entirely. By the age of 16 or 17, your young adult ought to be able to completely support themselves. Let them know this is what is expected of them and by 18 they should be ready to move out of the house to start their life.

From the age of 11, I either had some kind of job or was looking for one. I remember at 14yrs old caddying in the morning and pumping gas at night to earn enough money to go to baseball camp. By the time I was 17 I KNEW I no longer need financial support from my parents. At age 18 I moved out on my own and shared a 2 bedroom apt with three other people. This ability to hustle and earn money gave me tremendous confidence that still is with me today. Having your kids getting used to earning money and being independent and self-sufficient at a young age will do the same for them. Along with the myriad of life experiences work brings, the sense of liberation and confidence instilled in them is invaluable. Here are some of the many jobs I worked before the age of eighteen.

Paperboy, stock boy, caddy, car washer, gas station attendant, truck loader (in a meat freezer), mover, retail salesperson, short order cook, busboy, waiter, construction worker, truckdriver. I also would shovel driveways and mow lawns whenever the opportunity arose. Working will teach your children the value of money, the pride of putting in a good day's work and maybe how difficult life will be if you must work for someone else. Encourage your kids to be creative and wise, then maybe they will find a way to earn money that is temperamentally suitable for them. Maybe they can start their own business. A way to earn money that makes them feel useful and satisfied, a business that serves the world. It is very difficult to find work today that doesn't involve crime or compromise of one's integrity. Have your child begin to consider what they may want to do when they are full grown adults.

I would also recommend that you do not allow your grown kids to live in your house past the age of 18 unless they are paying close to a fair market rent. Even then, staying at home can be debilitating for them. There is a reason why the mama bird pushes their young out of the nest. If you want your kids to fly, force them to do so. It may be difficult for you but you will be grateful later. Let them know this is what is expected of them at age 9 or 10.

Changing the family diet

Parents are always asking "what about my kids, how should I feed them?" Obviously, there is a lot of confusion concerning the healthiest way to feed ourselves and our children. I cannot think of a better answer than to turn your attention once again to the natural world. Animals in the wild have NO confusion about what to feed their offspring. Every mammal nurses their young and when ready, the young ones begin to feed themselves, according to their natural instincts. Unfortunately, our natural instincts have been annihilated by salesmanship, propaganda, fear, ignorance, and greed.

It is imperative that you as a parent realize that keeping the peace in your home is more important than changing your (kids or spouse's) diets immediately (unless your child is seriously ill). Obviously, if you have one or two infants or very young children you can implement a diet change fairly easily. If your kids are older than 5 or 6 you are going to have to be more diplomatic. If you insist on taking something away (meat, dairy, soda, sugar, highly refined foods) you MUST have one or two viable and tasty substitutes.

First of all get a water purifier for your home that eliminates chlorine and fluoride, two highly toxic poisons that will cause disease. Get water purifiers for your shower heads as well so you are not showering with chlorine.

In most cases, the older your kids are the more difficult it will be for them. Be patient and don't force anything on your kids or your spouse. When you begin to make changes it is likely your family members will get interested in what you are doing and will see immediate improvements in your health, be it an immediate loss of fat, improved skin tone, brighter eyes and an increase in energy. (Once again it is nearly impossible to live on a raw food diet and be fat.)

If they are not interested you are better off leaving them alone. You can begin to educate them or have them read this book. Also find out what is important to them be it better skin, a leaner look, athletic prowess, increased energy and attention span etc. and let them know eating in this manner will get them what they want. Be Clever.

Here are some things you can do without much resistance. Replace all white sugar in the house with stevia or agave. Both are just as sweet as the poisonous white sugar but a much healthier option. You can replace salt shakers with "low sodium" salted seasonings, then move on to unsalted seasonings as time goes on. Try to rid your house of table salt and sea salt. Salt creates a lot of health problems including high blood pressure. Try Dulse (seaweed) flakes instead. You can replace milk with almond milk and you can also make raw ice cream by peeling bananas and freezing them. Put them in the blender or food processor when they soften a little blend them until creamy—it is delicious! Add berries, raw almond butter or tahini and you have an even tastier ice cream. You can replace unhealthy sugary popsicles by buying your own popsicle molds and using different mixtures of fresh coconut water, OJ, berries, mango, melon, grapes, strawberries, bananas etc. The kids love to invent their own popsicles. Replace the acid pasteurized juice in your fridge with freshly squeezed OJ, or freshly squeezed grapefruit juice. Most kids enjoy making juices. Tell them you'll "let them" help.

Giving your child soda and refined sugar is a form of child abuse. If you are already doing it you MUST wean them off. There are more "natural" sodas on the market if you have to give them soda. Explain to them that you have made a terrible mistake and that you are sorry. Do all you can to get them to drink freshly made juices. They will thank you one day. Remember all pasteurized juices are acidic and create stomach and teeth problems.

If your family members insist on bread make sure to buy whole grains instead of white bread. Remember the more refined a food is the more it will cause fat and disease. Since bread is very hard to digest it creates a lot of excess body fat and digestive problems. Also, many humans are allergic to gluten found in wheat products.

Try Manna bread or Essene bread. This is sprouted bread that is raw and/or barely cooked. It tastes delicious and digests much easier. Also, it is free of preservatives, salt, and refined sugar. You can find this bread in the freezer section of your health food store.

Instead of using dairy cheese, which is extremely disease producing, you can use Daiya (brand name) "cheese." Completely non-dairy, no soy and absolutely delicious. Daiya is a cooked food and I do not claim that it is health giving, but it is MUCH healthier than the normal cheese most people eat. Amy's (brand name) makes organic, dairy free, mac and cheese that can be purchased in the frozen section of your health food store or supermarket as well as many other tasty vegan dishes.

Replace sugared peanut butter with un-sugared peanut butter or almond butter and maybe even raw almond butter. Raw tahini is delicious as well. Raw nut butters are all healthy and taste great. Roasted nut butters are acidic and create health problems.

There are SO many vegan and vegetarian replacements for hamburgers and hot dogs. Give them 5 or 6 choices and let them decide what the replacement will be. I would suggest avoiding the ones with soy products, as they are simply not healthy. Soy and tofu are incredibly hard to digest. Avoid them. One of the best veggie burgers on the market are the Sunshine Burgers. They come in a few different flavors and varieties and are delicious.

Amy's Sonoma burgers are soy free and vegan and also very good. In fact, Amy's has many different vegan meals that are much healthier than what most people eat. Aim to create a cruelty-free home (don't eat the animals!). Replace highly sugared tomato sauces with natural organic ones that don't use refined sugars. Keep dates, raisins, raw almonds, raw cashews and pecans around for snacks. Let your kids make their own trail mixes.

Try to buy nothing but organic food.

Remember that inorganic dried fruit can sometimes contain sulfur dioxide, a highly toxic poison. NEVER let your family eat inorganic dried fruit if sulfur dioxide has been used.

Try your best to have your family start the day off with only fruit or fresh fruit juices. Fresh fruit salads are delicious, especially when you add bananas and raisins. Let the kids concoct their own fruit juices and smoothies and give a prize at the end of the week for "best juice maker."

There are also some great organic raw cereals and muesli on the market and using coconut water or almond milk with it is simply delicious. If you have raw almond butter you can simply put a spoon of it in the blender with water or coconut water and you will have instant almond milk.

Start every dinner off with a big salad (in hopes to soon have the entire dinner be a big salad), Challenge your family members to come up with the best healthiest salad and /or salad dressings. Give a prize, or special privileges to whoever comes up with the best salad, best dressing and/or the best raw dinner ideas. There are hundreds of ingredients to choose from; numerous lettuces and greens, sprouts, raisins, nuts (walnuts, pecans, almonds, macadamia,) seeds (sunflower, hemp, sesame) berries, Dulse flakes or leaves, and endless types of dressings you can make at home in a few minutes. Once you have everyone engaged it will get very fun! Avoid vinegar-laced salad dressings. Vinegar contains acetic acid which creates a lot of health problems. AVOID VINEGAR. Try Lemon Juice, Lime juice, Orange juice, Grapefruit juice as salad dressing.

Try to explain to them that you have just learned that most disease, cancer, obesity, heart disease, arthritis, osteoporosis, skin problems, acne, high blood pressure, clogged arteries diabetes etc. are caused by eating a denatured toxic diet. Tell them that if they learn how to eat correctly now they will have a huge advantage in life and can live with great energy and vitality their entire lives with no concern for disease or decrepitude. They also can avoid the deleterious effects of pharmaceutical drugs. Also that with time, the foods they once loved and are addicted to will no longer be appealing or even taste good, while fruits and vegetables will begin to taste better and better. Besides being healthier they will also save tens thousands of dollars by avoiding doctors and sick days at work. If this is not enough, try tailoring specific incentives for each family member to improve the quality of their food intake.

Kid's food addictions

Food addictions are very strong, especially those foods filled with salt and sugar. Tell them you have new foods to try . . . it may take a little time to get used to the newer healthier foods. Find out what is important to your kids. Tell them that eating like this is going to help them get what they want . . . Be straight with them. Being funny helps too. Try to introduce them to kids either online or in person who eat with consciousness. Give them this book to read and/or read it with them.

DO NOT cause prolonged tension and angst in your home. If family members are highly resistant then you must go easy. A peaceful home with a loving under-standing patient, parent is more important than having everyone convert right away. Obviously, if you have a child that is experiencing serious health problems you are going to have to get very creative in your approach.

The dinner table should be a place of joy and good humor. For too many children it is a nightmare of harsh-ness and inconsideration and bullying. This kind of behavior will create emotional problems around food that may last a lifetime.

Never force your child to eat.

This is a ridiculous practice of many parents who are impatient and short-sighted. There is no normal child that will starve themselves. If your child is not hungry why on earth would you force them to eat? Do you think if they miss a meal they will die? Or if they don't eat they will somehow be at a disadvantage? If your infant or child isn't hungry or doesn't want to eat do not yell at them or punish them.

Sometimes skipping a meal or two is just what the body needs. Offer them something else and/or tell them they can be excused. If there are foods they do not like do NOT force them to eat it as that is a cruel thing to do. If the lack of appetite continues you may want to inquire if there is some undue emotional stress going on. It is bound to happen that your baby or child will not want to eat at certain meal times. Do not force them or make them feel bad about it.

Some children are disgusted by certain foods, forcing them to eat those foods is abusive. Don't do it. How would you like to be forced to eat something that disgusts you?

Many life-long problems with your child's eating habits can be avoided by being conscientious, patient and loving. You should never force your child to eat anything. You can encourage, try to influence, coax, or even bribe them to try something, but do not force them as it can create anxiety, fear and abnormal behavior around food.

People often ask "what about birthday parties and family events where healthy eating is not a priority or even available?" That is a great question and seems unsolvable to many but simple solutions are extant. The fact is that children and families get together to be with each other. It just so happens that this usually includes plenty of food. Have your child eat a big meal before they arrive at the party so that they are not hungry when the party starts. You can also bring a meal with you and just let the host parent know that this is what your child will be eating during meal-time.

When everyone sits down to eat serve your child the food you brought. If you can serve it on the same kind of plates the other children have it will help. If you can get the same person that is serving the other children to serve your child that will also help draw less unwanted attention to your child. Be discreet about it. Do not make a big deal about the food and nobody else will. You can also bring snacks and a fruit, or coconut shake, raisins, dried mangoes, nuts etc. for later in the party. When cake is served you can give your child a piece of a raw pie that you made or bought. Ask your child what is important to them about the party and what they would like to happen when it's time to eat and when the cake comes. If you have a strategy together there will be no issues at all.

School

No matter how good or great your school system is, you should never relinquish full responsibility to an institution. You are their parent and YOU are responsible for their education. Many of our school's requirements and curriculum are filled with nonsense, deception and a boat full of lies and propaganda. History and science books are so fraught with misinformation, exaggerations, ignorance, and half-truths, that those who are good students have learned mostly lies. Please read *Dumbing Us Down* by John Taylor Gatto.

Homeschooling your child is the best choice to make and it is a movement on the rise here in America. There are many sources and organizations that will help and support you in this wonderful endeavor. You will be amazed at how fast your child will learn and how much more efficient and intelligent this system is compared to the school system in place.

All any child wants to do is learn. However, they all learn differently and at a different pace. It doesn't make one "smarter" because they learn faster or "dumber" because they learn slower. As a parent, the best thing you can do is see what your child is interested in and teach them all they want to learn about the subject at home. No matter what subject it is, there are many ways to learn and teach about it. Also, teaching a young child about something you are interested in can be wonderful as well. Whether it is baseball or quantum physics a shared interest provides fertile ground for learning and expanding the mind and imagination as well as deepening your relationship with your child. Try to use books and discussions for teaching. Avoid computers and screens as much as possible.

It can be a lot of fun to introduce your child to activities that you enjoy. Often times your child may like the same activities that you do and that can be a really wonderful thing to share. However, it is vital that you do not live through your child or force them into activities just because YOU like them. This behavior creates a lot of resentment and hatred and makes the child feel like they are responsible for your happiness. See what constructive activities they like and encourage them to do it. If they are disinterested in what you love, move on. Do not impose yourself on the child. That is selfish, immature and very damaging.

Many parents today are insisting that their children become highly accomplished scholars, athletes, musicians or "geniuses." What I have seen from these types of parents is quite frightening and very sad. Their child is no longer a child with their own unique thoughts feelings and desires but only a tool for the insistent parent to mold into THEIR idea of a "success." It is cruel and dehumanizing. This IS a form of abuse as the child loses his/her ability to make any choices or fulfill their own wishes.

It is one thing when you have a child who has a genuine passion for an activity and VOLUNTARILY puts their heart and soul into the activity. That can be wonderful and it is only a boon to the child if the parent supports them and helps them in that endeavor.

All too often a child is given no chance to choose but forced and bullied by the parent to become "great" at the activity despite the fact that the child may have little or no interest. It is hard for many parents to separate themselves from their children but also quite necessary. Allowing your child to find THEIR passion is much more effective than trying to force your passion on them. Your only insistence ought to be that they develop a strong character, do their best, have a sense of decency and goodwill towards others. If you can give them that then you will both be successful.

It is a great idea to expose your children to as many activities as possible and see what they gravitate towards. Be patient it may take many years before they find what they love.

Allow your child to follow his or her impulses, as long as it doesn't hurt anyone or damage valuable property. If your child wants to draw on the wall, designate a spot for just that. If your child wants to take all the pots and pans out and spread them out on the floor, allow it. Why not join them? It makes a great drum set and is easy to clean up. If your child wants to "build a fort" in the living room . . . help them. Build the best fort ever! They will always remember it. If your child wants to sing a song really loud allow them. (If after a while it is getting to you try this: Begin to sing with them just as loud for about a minute. Then start singing in a quieter manner. Then even quieter so it is a whisper-soft song. Eventually, they will be singing so softly it will not disturb you. You can also just sing along with them until they tire out.

Childhood illness

"Normal" childhood diseases such as mumps, chicken pox, measles, rubella, ear infections, whooping cough, asthma, constipation, acne, diabetes and all types of flu simply do not exist for the child that is eating exclusively raw fruits, vegetables, seeds, and nuts. Even children who eat 80% raw food and are vegans will avoid most or all of these "normal diseases."

Despite a very clean diet your child may still experience mild sickness, this could be for many different reasons. Your child may still get sick from a high dose of toxins in the air, emotional turmoil, lack of proper sleep and/or exposure to cold. Obviously, try to keep your child warm when it is cold out and if your child does develop a cough and/or a fever, simply keep them warm (especially head and feet) and let them rest. Fresh orange juice is a big help along with a lot of love and attention. They will usually be better in a day or two.

Medication is never necessary to return your child back to health and is always dangerous. Commonly dispensed antibiotics are very dangerous and cause all kinds of further problems down the road (re-read Chapters 4 and 5). Rest, fresh orange juice and a lot of love will always do the trick. Of course, if your child has had a long and serious history of health problems and has been taking medicine constantly, you may want to slowly wean them off the drugs as their health increases through a proper diet.

If your child has a temperature, which is quite common, as the skin is the number one pathway to release toxins . . . monitor it closely and never allow it to go over 103 degrees. If it does (which is Very rare) begin to put ice on the child's neck and forehead to bring the temperature down. Or place the child in a cool bath. Never allow a temperature of 104 degrees or more.

ADHD

Behavior will immediately improve on a natural diet. ADHD is a ridiculous, fictitious, made up "disease" to make the incredibly rich and powerful pharmaceutical companies more rich and powerful. It is right up there with "restless leg syndrome" and "binge eating disorder" in the absurdity arena. Drug companies will do all they can to ensnare potential customers and turn them into pharmaceutical drug addicts, including creating a diagnosable "disease" out of the most ordinary human behaviors. According to statistics from the CDC "the annual societal 'cost of illness' for ADHD is estimated to be between $36 and $52 billion, in 2005 dollars." Of course, these profits are ever increasing as "awareness" (Promotion) that kids who have difficulty paying attention are not, in fact, normal but have a "disease" that must be "treated" with drugs.

"ADHD *is fraud intended to justify starting children on a life of drug addiction,*" said Dr. Edward C. Hamlyn, a founding member of the Royal College of General Practitioners, back in 1998 about the phony condition.

We all know that a "life of drug addiction" for the now more than 3 million children in this country who are given Ritalin and Adderal. This means billions of dollars for drug companies, I couldn't agree more with Dr. Hamlyn. Do you think the pharmaceutical companies care more about your child's well being than they do about profits?

The symptoms of ADHD according to the CDC: People with ADHD show a persistent pattern of inattention and/or hyperactivity-impulsivity that interferes with functioning or development:

1. Inattention: Six or more symptoms of inattention for children up to age 16, or five or

more for adolescents 17 and older and adults; symptoms of inattention have been present for at least 6 months, and they are inappropriate for developmental level:

- Often fails to give close attention to details or makes careless mistakes in schoolwork, at work, or with other activities.
- Often has trouble holding attention to tasks or play activities.
- Often does not seem to listen when spoken to directly.
- Often does not follow through on instructions and fails to finish schoolwork, chores, or duties in the workplace (e.g., loses focus, side-tracked).
- Often has trouble organizing tasks and activities.
- Often avoids, dislikes, or is reluctant to do tasks that require mental effort over a long period of time (such as schoolwork or homework).
- Often loses things necessary for tasks and activities (e.g. school materials, pencils, books, tools, wallets, keys, paperwork, eyeglasses, mobile telephones).
- Is often easily distracted
- Is often forgetful in daily activities.

These are not medical symptoms! These are very common behaviors among children of all ages, especially boys. Any of these can be remedied by any thoughtful, patient parent who is willing to put in the time and effort to do so instead of numbing their kids on drugs.

Television and video games, a poor heavily sugared and processed diet are a sure way to guarantee your child has a short attention span and a lazy mind.

A staggering 10 million children in the United States are being prescribed addictive stimulants, antidepressants, and other psychotropic (mind-altering) drugs for these so-called educational and behavioral problems. This is a drug company initiated, national epidemic and disaster that few are even aware of.

According to IMS Health Vector One National database, from April 2014:

> 274,804 INFANTS were taking psychiatric drugs. 370,778 from ages 2–3, 600,948 from ages 4–5 and close to 8,000,000 from 6 to 17. According to the *New York Times*, some 83,000 prescriptions for Prozac were given to children under the age of 2 in 2014. Risperdal is a medication prescribed to infants and toddlers. It is an antipsychotic intended to treat schizophrenia and bipolar disorder. How outrageous that drug companies, doctors, and parents not only allow this to go on but actually endorse and promote it. These drugs are dangerous mind-altering entities that can cause severe damage and real mental illness. Any informed parent can avoid ALL of this madness.

Teaching your child to read and reading with them and to them is a guarantee that their attention span will be better than average. Discussing what you are reading will get their mind engaged and create the ability to express themselves. You can learn so much about your child by the way in which they interpret stories.

Playing Chess, learning a musical instrument and athletic activity will also increase their ability to concentrate. Teaching them how to draw, or simply allowing them to create a piece of art with an aim in mind will develop their ability to concentrate. Gently nudge your young child to finish their work. It is a good habit to get used to.

Learning any athletics such as gymnastics, swimming, basketball, football, baseball, track, martial arts, boxing, skating, skateboarding, tennis, golf, and dance also will give your child an ability to focus and develop concentration. (It is imperative to teach your child to swim for safety's sake and children really love to play in the water with their parents.)

The only "solutions" modern medicine has are surgeries and pharmaceutical drugs. Most surgeries are completely unnecessary. The drugs are a Disaster. These drugs have "side effects" or as I more accurately like to call them DIRECT FRONTAL ASSAULTS on your health and the health of your child.

Medical diagnoses are so often wrong. *There is no such thing as an accurate diagnosis for a made up disease.* Allowing a doctor's opinion to determine the possibilities for your child and their life is Dangerous. There are Thousands of stories of doctors claiming a child (or adult)is incapable of having a normal life due to some condition or disease that they deem "incurable," and it turns out that because the parents insisted on investigating and experimenting the child goes on to have an extraordinary and drug-free life.

Raun Kaufman was born with what doctors called "severe autism."

He did not respond to the outside world at all. Raun's parents were told that he had an "I.Q. of 30" and would not be able to have a normal life. The "treatments" available to him by the medical world were heavy drugging regimes; behavioral training where physical punishment was involved and other acts of inhumanity. Raun's parents Barry and Samarhia decided that they were going to decline on the available "treatments." They took responsibility for their son and decided that they would completely accept and love this "mentally disabled" child. Instead of forcing their world onto him, they decided that they would enter into his world.

So when the boy would flap his hands, rock his body, or spin plates for hours and hours at a time different family members would do it with him. Instead of forcing him to learn what was "acceptable" behavior and judging him as "slow" or "undeveloped," they completely accepted him. As time went on there would be moments of the boy responding to his outside world, taking in others and recognizing their presence. Something that never happened before.

Raun's parents also changed his diet, removing dairy products and refined foods.

To make a long and glorious story short, Raun made a complete recovery with a near genius IQ and Graduated with a degree from Brown University in Bio-medical ethics.

The story was made into a book and a movie called *Son Rise*. The Kaufmans run a center in Massachusetts called Autism Treatment Center of America for parents and their children who have been diagnosed with this "incurable disease." Scores and scores of children given no hope have gone on to lead normal and extraordinary lives.

This is definitely true for Jacob Barnett, the 17-year-old young man who was diagnosed as "autistic," whose mother was told that her son would probably never read or write. Today, Jacob is a genius already working on his Master's Degree in quantum physics while most of his peers are still in junior high. He is also currently developing his own original theory in astrophysics, according to recent reports.

You can go to youtube and see both Raun and Jacob being interviewed.

They are extremely intelligent and well developed young men.

According to the medical world, not one child has ever recovered from Autism (thus the label "incurable"). In plain language, their "treatments" do not work . . . ever. Yet most of the parents of "autistic" children follow doctors orders and give up on these children and/or drug them for the rest of their lives. Why? That means out of the millions they have treated not ONE has recovered.

ADHD is a fictitious disease. Your son or daughter can learn to change their behavior and thinking patterns by consistent efforts at new ways of thinking and feeling. Of course, proper feeding, mental training (reading, chess, music, ballet, gymnastics etc.) and a consistent physical regime will be a tremendous help.

Other than Cancer, Heart Disease, Osteoporosis, and Diabetes . . . There are few medical diagnoses that are meaningful. ALL of these just mentioned diseases have been and continue to be reversed without ANY drugs. There is SO much misunderstanding and so many false beliefs regarding these medical diagnoses. Be very wary of ANY medical diagnosis concerning you or your child, especially "behavioral diseases" or conditions. Paying attention and staying focused are skills that can be learned and developed.

Closing thoughts on raising your child

A loving, intelligent parent will teach: Character is more important than anything, ANY problem can be solved, it is important to be resourceful and capable of earning money but money is not the most important thing. Fame is an illusion that never lasts and is always packaged with compromise and sorrow. Trying to "stay safe" can be very dangerous and stunt the spirit. ANY position of "power" usually requires significant compromises of your character. True power is being a sane, independent, capable, decent, loving, human being with a strong character and a desire to help others.

You do not own your child. You are the Guardian (you are to guard the child against baneful influence and harmful people and activities) you are the parent, NOT the owner. If you remember this you will treat your child with the proper respect and attitude. You will remember that your child has his/her own individual thoughts and feelings that may not match yours. That is not only ok, it is natural. Do NOT take it personally. Do not force your child to "follow in your footsteps," or try to live out some fantasy or picture you have in your head of what they should be. That will only cause resentment and pain all around. Try to expose them to as many interests and activities as possible and see what they gravitate towards. Certainly encourage them, cheer them on and support them. Explain to them and/or demonstrate that hard work and mindful practice pays off. The more accepting and patient you are towards your child, the more you will allow them to grow and the more respect and love they will have for you. Forcing your child into any activity whether it be football or piano is violent. Every child loves something and it is your job to find out what that is.

Treat your child with respect, listen and watch. Be the kind of person you wish your child to be. Children will not always do as you say but often will do as you do. The early years of a child's development are filled with imitation. If you show high standards, patience, goodwill, courage, honesty, fine manners, humor, decency and morality they will copy you. They will also copy your poor behavior as well. Be careful.

Your child will fall down . . . a lot, literally, and figuratively. You can teach them to laugh it off as 99% of the time they fall they will not be seriously hurt. When you fall laugh, get up, brush yourself off and keep going. Teach this to your children. Adapting the same attitude when you fall, make a mistake or are involved in a blunder will be a great example for them. Learn to laugh it off and keep going. Many children cry from the shock of the fall and often continue crying for no good reason. This often becomes a bad habit.

You will be amazed at the results if, when your child first starts to walk, you instill this idea that a fall in and of itself is no reason to cry but a very good reason to laugh. Laugh with them every time they fall (preferably on the grass or a soft carpet.) Teaching them to laugh off minor scrapes, cuts, and bruises in the physical realm will also carry over to the many disappointments they will face in life.

Of course that 1% of the time when your child has really taken a hard fall, it is wise to comfort and hold the child until the crying stops. Physical contact and hugs are soothing at these times. Even in these instances, there are lessons that can be learned and ways to help your child get through the pain. Use humor. "That blood belongs on the inside! What is it doing out here?" Ask your child where it hurts and gently put your hand on that place, to comfort your child. When you see an opening, ask your child "Can I just smack your leg really hard? That way you'll forget about the pain in your elbow?" "Let me pinch you really hard right here and you'll forget about that bruised knee!" This will often bring laughter to a small child and that can be a big help, as it is impossible to be in pain while in the throes of laughter. I am not suggesting for you to be flippant but I am suggesting that distractions and humor along with love and affection can be a great relief. Pretending to hurt yourself often makes a child laugh as well.

All children, no matter what age, should learn how to swim and be able to survive in the water for at least

10 minutes without holding on to anything. The sooner they learn this the better. If you do not know how to swim learn with them and make it fun. Kids love the water and will love it more if they are proficient at swimming. (Search YouTube for "babies learning to swim.")

All children (Girls and Boys) should learn how to defend themselves. Boxing and Martial Arts are very effective. If you have no self-defense training, take classes or lessons with your child. (Kids love a punching bag and it is a good idea to have one in the house.) Make sure their teacher is of a high character and competent. If they don't love it explain to them that it is necessary and try to make it as fun as possible. Offer a reward for their participation. Yes, bribery works.

Spend at least one or two hours a day reading to your children. Make sure there is always a bedtime story before they go to sleep.

Reading expands your child's imagination, focus, intelligence, patience, ability to communicate and can propel your child to a very rich and wonderful life. A well-told story can stay with your child forever and inspire them throughout their lives. Read at a young age, certain stories will imprint on your child's memory, values and ways of thinking that can shape their lives and provide guidance and assurance during difficult times. Give them a choice each night between two or three different books. Let them pick if they want to.

Do your best to keep your children screen free (TV, Phones, Tablets, video games etc).

Religion and your child

It is useful to teach your child that there is a Supreme Being and a Creator and/or creative force or God. I think it is absurd to believe that a huge explosion or an accidental, random "big bang" created an eyeball or a brain cell or formed a tree, and created the stars. I do not believe that such precise and intricate creations "happened" by a random accident. No man created and designed a heart or an ear drum. It appears something greater does exist.

Teaching your child a specific religion can be a slippery slope. Religion seems a lot like fire. Fire can save your life, keep you warm and comfortable in the freezing cold but can also burn you to death. Millions of religious people find useful guidance through their practice and devotion that helps them build and maintain a value system that is an obvious boon to society. Many churches, synagogues, and mosques are a strong source of support for their communities and provide excellent services. The sense of community, living according to certain standards and values, belief in a higher being and the many charitable acts that places of worship and their organizations provide have helped and continue to help millions of people.

I have also seen religious organizations become the cause of great fear, pain, suffering and massive confusion . . . even violence and wars. Some religious sects have a mind controlling, cult-like quality to them that does nothing but crush the true essence and individuality of the participant.

Religious fanatics, along with New Age Charlatans are a dime a dozen and VERY dangerous people. So this is a tough question you may want to seriously consider. You may want to ask yourself a few questions. Do you want your child to be able to pick a religion or do you want it forced upon them? Do you want your child to be indoctrinated? Do you want your child to understand the origins of all Religions or just one? Do you want your child to understand that having no religion is just fine? Do you want to let your child know that many decent, loving responsible people have no religious practice at all? That some people do not even believe that there is a God or a supreme being and yet they live exemplary lives?

Have you ever changed your mind about something important? If so, is it possible that you may switch religions or give up your religious practices at some time in the near future and would you allow your child to switch as well? If your religion confuses you or has caused you pain and confusion, why teach it to your child?

I would suggest discussing the magnificent creations that surround us on a daily basis. Trees, plant life, the myriad of beautiful and astonishing animals, the sky, the ocean and rivers and all the beings that live underwater. Discuss the wonder of it all with your child and do your best not to impose religious beliefs but maybe ask a lot of questions to your child . . . and yourself about how all this came to be. Skip the dogma and the judgment and harshness of many religious beliefs.

It is an important thing to allow your child to form their own beliefs and to provide your child with as much information and experience you can provide them. Many children want to please their parents and will often simply adhere to what is being taught externally but may be severely conflicted and or confused internally. Mechanically repeating prayers and rituals that have no personal meaning is not helping your child develop. Believing in things that they have no understanding about creates conflict. Living in fear of a punishing God creates undue fear and pressure and being ashamed about their natural desires creates a lot of dysfunctional behavior. Please be wary of your wish to impose your religious beliefs on your child. Consider that your child has a mind of their own and they will do much better if their mind is not filled with superstition and strange teachings.

CULT AWARENESS

America and the rest of the world need to begin to educate our children and the adult population on the dangers of cults and cult mind control. Each year Millions of people around the world join cults. Some of these cults are extremely harsh and demand full control of their devotees. Many lives have been destroyed by these mind control groups. Please educate yourself and your children on this matter. Even the most highly educated and the most brilliant people have been sucked into mind control groups. Please do not think your child is immune from the possibility of being victimized.

According to *Psychology Today* and Dr. Adrian Furnham:

> There is a great deal of interest in cults which can take many forms. They may be religious or

racial, political or mystical, self-help or pseudo-psychological, but they all have half a dozen recognizable characteristics:

—Powerful and exclusive devotion to a particular person or creed.

—The use of "thought reform" programs to integrate, socialize, persuade and therefore control members.

—A well thought through recruitment, selection and socialization process.

—Attempts to maintain psychological and physical dependency among cult members.

—Cults insist on reprogramming the way people see the world.

—Consistent exploitation of group members specifically to advance the leaders goals.

—Ultimately using Psychological and physical harm to cult members, their friends and relatives and possibly the community as a whole.

Please educate yourself and your family members about this dangerous phenomenon.

Steven Hassan has written a couple of excellent books on this subject called Combating Mind Control and Freedom of Mind. One serious, informed discussion on this subject can help you and your loved ones avoid a disastrous situation.

BOOKS

Required reading for parents

Ina May's Guide To Childbirth, Ina May Gaskin
Natural Childbirth the Bradley Way, Susan McCutcheon
Dr. Linda Palmer Baby Matters
Dumbing us Down, John Taylor Gatto
Mister Rodgers Parenting Book, Fred Rodgers
Confessions of a Medical Heretic, Dr. Robert Mendelsohn
The Tavistock Institute, David Estulin
Propaganda, Edward Bernays
Consolation of Philosophy, Boethius
Meditations, Marcus Aurelius
Essays, Ralph Waldo Emerson
Raising Your Child From Before Birth To Maturity, this
    book is contained in "The Art Of Personality"
    Hazrat Inayat Khan.
Bronson Alcott Peabody Diary of a School
People's History of America, Howard Zinn
Siddartha, Herman Hesse
Tragedy and Hope, Carrol Quigley

Required videos for parents

The Ultimate History Lesson, John Taylor Gatto
Mr. Rogers Talks With Parents About Discipline
Vaxxed—from Cover Up to Catastrophe
Bought—the movie
The Men Who Own and Run the US Government

The Tavistock Institute—Interview with Dr. John Coleman.
The Hobart Shakespeareans
50-year-old recording explains why the world is falling apart.
Trophy Kids

Books for kids

Dr. Seuss, *Cat in the Hat, The Lorax, Oh The Places You'll Go*, etc.
The Wizard of Oz
King Arthur
All books by Hans Christian Anderson
Little Women
Short stories by Louisa May Alcott
Adventures of Tom Sawyer
Huckleberry Finn
Oliver Twist
A Christmas Carol
Little House in the Big Woods (Laura Ingalls Wilder)
Grimms Brothers Fairy Tales (unedited)
Aesops Fables
Herman Hess Fairy Tales
Dear America (book series)
Where the Red Fern Grows.
The Secret Garden
Matilda
The Wind in the Willows
Madeline

The House at Pooh Corner
The Story of Ferdinand
Charlotte's Web
I Capture the Castle
A Wrinkle in Time
Mixed-up Files of Mrs. Basil E. Frankweiler
The Invention of Hugo Cabret
The Little Prince
Matilda
The Phantom Tollbooth
Roll of Thunder Hear my Cry
Bullfinches Mythology
The Odyssey
The Illiad
Sophocles Plays
Shakespeare's Plays

Movies can be educational, uplifting and very entertaining. However, books induce your child to use their imagination and minds in ways that movies and television shows do not. Get your child in the habit of Reading at a very early age and avoid all screen time for as long as you can. By the age of 6 or 7, you can begin to slowly introduce them to watching movies. I would suggest one movie night per week until they are teenagers.

Recommended movies

Sound of Music
Wizard of Oz

Little Women
My Fair Lady
Oliver Twist
Mary Poppins
Heidi
The Lorax
Babe
Where The Red Fern Grows
It's a Wonderful Life
Singin' in the Rain
Oh God
Up
Annie
The Kid (Chaplin)
Home Alone
The Black Stallion
Back To The Future
Mother Ocean
Stand By Me
The Princess Bride
Matilda
The Karate Kid
Big
To Kill A Mockingbird
Inside Out
Hunger Games Series

TV series

(Available on YouTube)

Little House on the Prairie
Highway to Heaven
Mr. Rodgers Neighborhood
The Muppet Show
The Waltons
The Wonder Years
Lassie
Flipper
(just for laughs)
Charlie Chaplin movies
Bugs Bunny
The Little Rascals

Websites

Alliance For Natural health: anh-usa.org
Naturalparentsnetwork.com
Globalresearch.org
Vactruth.com
mercola.com
Anticorruptionsociety.com
The Power of Natural Healing Radio Show, Howard
    Strauss.
gerson.org

Do your best to keep your children screen free (TV,
Phones, Tablets, video games etc).

Some thoughts on feeding your pets.

Remember that nature doesn't lie or propagandize. NO animals in nature eat cooked food. No one can argue that fact. I have had two dogs of my own and they have both thrived on a mostly raw/vegetarian diet. I have a 15-year old dog right now that looks like she is about 7 years old . . . and no botox! I would never feed my pet dog food. If you knew the ingredients of most dog foods you would decline as well. My dogs love/d; carrots, apples, avocado, bananas, cantaloupe, mango, walnuts, cashews, macadamia nuts, dates, almond butter and rarely turned down any vegan treat cooked or raw. They have loved potatoes, cauliflower, broccoli, brussel sprouts, pasta, bread etc.

I have never raised a cat. I have had friends who have raised their cats on nothing but raw food. (Look up "Pottenger's cats") I have been told that cats need to eat meat and that makes sense to me. These cats did eat raw meat but just a few times a week and were exceptionally healthy. They enjoyed wheatgrass, some vegetables, and chicken gizzards. I am not an animal expert but there are many websites you can refer to. Google "raw food cats." AND you always have your common sense and ability to observe the natural world.

SOME NOTES
ON MY RECOVERY

Here is a brief overview of my experience of being very sick and regaining health.

I remember standing and waiting for the elevator in my building to arrive. The next thing I knew, I was falling. I hit the ground, right shoulder first. I was very confused. I did not pass out, yet I did not know I was falling. I had completely lost my balance without ANY neurological feedback from my body or brain. A building employee ran to help me. No serious bodily damage but I knew I was in deep trouble physically. Things just went downhill from there.

At my worst, I had little or no feeling from my chest down. Most of my body was numb. I was extremely fatigued, despite the fact I would sleep for 12 or 14 hours. My lower body felt as if it were in constant spasm, and it was. I actually could see muscles constantly twitching throughout my upper and lower leg without any intention on my part to do so. I hardly had an appetite and my digestive system all but shut down. I had occasional spasms on my face and some extreme hypersensitivity in my feet. My eyes would sometimes go into a brief spasm. I was unable to move my legs without using my arms to move them around. I could not stand. I could use my hands but they were desensitized and debilitated. My manual dexterity was about 40% and I was unable to hold a guitar pick; as soon as I struck the strings it fell from my hands. Nor could I coordinate my left hand to touch the strings I wanted to touch. Needless to say, I was depressed, angry, and impatient.

I had been a highly competitive athlete my whole life and all of a sudden I was a cripple. I was shocked, scared, and embarrassed. I didn't want anyone to see me in this condition. I'll never forget the first day I went out of my building being pushed in my wheelchair. I remember the look on the faces of my neighbors of shock and disbelief. Some of them literally couldn't speak and I realized then just how awful I must look to evoke such a reaction. Rumours had spread that I had been shot or in a car accident I weighed about 160 lbs, down from a very trim and fit 190lbs. For seven months I was in this completely debilitated state.

The fact was, my body was breaking down and all I was interested in was regaining my health. That's it. I refused to use any medical terminology to describe my condition and when friends and family would emphatically ask me "what is it?" or "what did the doctors say?" I would repeat, "I'm not interested in what the doctors

say; I'm interested in regaining my health." The manner
in which medicine names disease is racked with recklessness, inaccuracies, and little or no science. The diagnosis
also carries with it the prognosis. Prognosis is the nar-
row-minded OPINION of what the outcome will be.
It does not take into account ANY of the intangibles of
what a person is made up of. It also directly limits many
patients possibilities, especially those that 'believe in their
doctor.'

I saw at least 15–20 different doctors in seven
months. This was not by choice. If it were up to me I
would have gladly stayed home. I had fallen behind on
my rent, and the landlord was threatening to kick me out.
I had to go to the hospital to get insurance forms filled
out to prove I was sick to help me pay my rent, as I obviously couldn't work.

It was bad enough that I had to have doctors examine me, poke and prod me, despite the fact I simply wasn't
going to take any medication. Secretly I wished that one
of them would come up with something that would prove
helpful to me, that didn't happen. For a couple of weeks,
they wanted to inject my spine with a radioactive fluid
and then x-ray my spine. I refused. They got angry. They
could not understand why I, in such a debilitated state,
wouldn't adhere to their protocol. They literally thought
I was insane but the point was "I don't believe in any of
your treatments, in fact I know them to be toxic, dangerous and would only cause me more physical problems.
You doctors yourselves can report only in the best case
scenarios, a 'mild' improvement with these treatments
and in only a few cases. I am not interested in a mild

improvement nor in the shocking range and depth of 'side-effects' that come hand in hand with these treatments. On top of that I prefer to have the radioactive liquid NOT in my bloodstream, thank you.

One time, at St. Luke's hospital, after being examined the doctors told me "we are going to have to admit you." I understood they wanted to help me and on this particular visit I was at my lowest or weakest point. Close to death is not at all an exaggeration. Three or four of the doctors and two or three of the nurses stood in a semi-circle before me as I sat in my wheelchair ready to leave. They insisted that I stay. It was a very poignant moment in my life that I will never forget. These men and women in their white coats, standing shoulder to shoulder trying to convince me to stay. Me, barely sitting up in my chair, physically exhausted, emotionally spent and just a couple more hopeful thoughts in my head. I wished they had something for me. I really did. I knew they didn't and began pushing my wheels and rolling forward as my chair approached them they parted and I wondered if I had sealed my fate for the worse or for the better. It may have been a foolish move or it may have saved my life. I sincerely thanked them for their effort and left the hospital.

What was worse than the visits, were the actual trips back and forth to the hospital. I was wheeled through my building to the elevator out to a waiting van that carried about four or five other wheelchair-bound patients. It was humiliating to be wheeled past neighbors and friends. I was pushed up a ramp into the van and they strapped the chair to the floor of the van while all this was happening I felt the dread of being helpless like never before. If the attendant made a mistake while loading or unloading the chair into the van I could easily have come off the ramp and have fallen to the ground and there was nothing I could do about it. It was very depressing. These men were competent but I had never had this experience and the speed at which they moved us was a little alarming, to say the least. I felt like cargo, not like a human being. It was depressing and dehumanizing. Nothing was said to those of us in the back of the van. I tried to speak to others but I don't remember much of a response. Nobody talked. It seemed as if they were lifeless, dead. I had to tuck my head down from hitting the roof as we rode through the bumpy streets of Manhattan. It felt like a prison atmosphere and frankly, we were prisoners. I was constantly planning my escape.

These doctors told me many different things, they were all trying to help, but I simply wasn't interested in their treatments. I refused all treatments and took none of the recommended drugs. The doctors had little hope for me ever recovering and a couple of them even suggested that I sign up with a handicap employment agency. I was handed the handicapped employment package on two different occasions. I gave it right back to them.

Not one doctor asked me about my life, what was going on emotionally, or intellectually. Not one.

I have to mention that while most people around me believed I would not get better, I KNEW would get better. It was only a matter of time. In fact, I actually looked at those people who thought I had no chance of recovery with utter astonishment, impatience, and anger. "Are you out of your mind?" "You do not know me." I would think and often say out loud. "There is NO WAY I'm staying in this present condition. NO WAY."

Whenever there was an inkling of doubt in my head It was replaced with the powerful life wish that burned in my gut, to get back to health.

I knew I had abused my body by overtraining, over-eating and lack of proper rest. In addition, I also had a strong sense that what I was experiencing in my body was also exacerbated caused by my emotional and mental state. I had always prided myself on not being addicted to any kind of drugs or alcohol. Little did I know there is a whole world of addictive behaviors that include neither one. I was an addict of another sort. Just before I was stricken, I went 36 weeks training three hours per day of highly intense weightlifting. I remember going weeks without a day off. I used the training as a way to deal with unmanageable emotions. The workouts left me physically exhausted and provided some temporary relief from the inner turmoil. The same way an alcoholic would drink to "feel better." The frequency and intensity of this program was certainly a shock to my nervous system. I was eating six times a day, which put a huge strain on my digestive system. I was sleeping five hours a night, giving lectures on medical fraud, hosting a cable television show, training five to six people a day. I was frightened of a quiet moment and would do anything not to face myself. I was angry, resentful, and eventually frightened at the condition of the world. Ironically, my inner world was what needed attention and I was completely focused on the outer world.

I didn't understand why people wouldn't listen to protocols of health that were tried and tested. I had seen people recover from serious illnesses and then go back to their old ways and die. I thought it was my fault. I couldn't understand why certain people would immediately take on these principles and get well and others would not. I actually believed that soon everyone would know about and believe in these concepts of health and healing and that the world would change. That the masses would understand these principles of health and stop looking for a pill to "make them well."

As Chuang-Tse, a student of Lao-Tsu author of The Tao says: "Great Truths do not Take Hold of the Masses."

It appears to me now that I was trying to save the world. That's always a tricky little role to play. What I really needed to do was save myself from the strange and unrealistic ideas and expectations I had.

Life gets very simple when you are unable to walk. Activity is limited and one can only watch so much television before the mind begins to cry for mercy. I could read for a couple of hours, but then my eyes would give out. At the early stages of my body's breakdown, I began to seek some help with my emotional life. The more severe my symptoms became, the more serious I got about my inner-work. I got involved in a 12 step program to help me deal with my addictive behaviors and harmful or toxic thought patterns.

This opened up a whole new world of self-responsibility for me, and at the same time was very difficult. I felt

"Anger: an acid that can do more harm to the vessel in which it is stored than to anything on which it is poured."

≋✲ LUCIUS ANNAEUS SENECA (4 BC–65 CE), ROMAN PHILOSOPHER AND PLAYWRIGHT the key to my recovery was in my heart and mind and I worked this program with great determination.

I made concerted efforts to examine my belief systems and see myself as I really was, not how I preferred to see myself. This was quite shocking, as I had always thought of myself as an easy-going, light-hearted, fun guy. In fact, I was dealing with a myriad of emotions from anger and resentment to bitterness and hate. On a suggestion, I began writing letters to friends, and family members saying exactly what I felt. I never sent these letters, as that was not the intent. By writing down on paper my thoughts and feelings I saw more clearly the depths of my anger. It was my responsibility to deal with this anger, stop blaming others and begin to gain some understanding of myself.

"When anger rises think of the consequences."

≡✲ CONFUCIUS
(551BC–479BC)

I know a lot of people think that anger is purely an emotional issue and that its effects on the physical body are limited. The fact is that people sometimes die in moments of extreme anger, as the blood pressure soars and the strain on the heart is sometimes too much. Usually, this occurs in a short and explosive outburst, but how many of us have ever considered the long-term effects of internal anger on the body? My experience is that being angry and resentful is the equivalent of taking poison and hoping somebody else dies.

I also noticed an increasing amount of fear in my life. Fear that the world was simply a horrible place that just kept getting worse, corrupt warmongering governments, rapacious corporations, and a "health care system" responsible for at least 300,000 deaths per year. I had thoughts that soon they would be coming for me as I often went on long tirades on my television show about the way things really operate. Having my phone tapped didn't help. We all know that human beings can, in fact, be scared to death if the fright is sudden and intense. Once again the question must be asked what are the long-term effects of living in fear? Can fear, over a period of time, steal nerve energy and life force? I think so.

The worse I got the harder I worked on these issues. I began to see clearly how much help I needed and I did something I hadn't done my entire life—I asked for help. This was very humbling to a man who had never asked for help. Nonetheless, I received help and began some practices that changed my life.

I began meditating every morning. At first, for 15 minutes a day and eventually, working my way up to 2 hours a day. During my meditation, I would take time to just sit and breathe, doing my best to quiet my run-on mind. I would practice sitting and observing the thoughts as they passed, doing my best not to identify with them, realizing that most of what I was "thinking" were random thoughts that just happened to be passing through the air. It was quite a revelation to recognize that I didn't choose to think them. It was vital to take this practice into the rest of the day I did my best to realize that I am not my thoughts and I can choose what I want to think. I could choose to go to heaven or hell with the thoughts I identified with. The idea was to take the experience of separation from my thoughts into my day.

I also spent many hours visualizing myself in my healthiest state, and recalling what it felt like to walk and run and be athletic. If you have any doubt whether this works or not try this experiment: Stand up and square off facing a wall. Pick up one hand directly in front of you to shoulder height. Your arm is parallel to the floor, your hand at shoulder height. Now take the straightened arm around behind you as far as you can like a hand on a clock. Do Not move your feet. When you can twist no more notice precisely notice where the arm is pointing. (On a 360-degree scale most people will get it back to 170 to 190 degrees.)

Now you are going to do it again this time, with some preparation. Continue to stand and face the wall with your arms by your side. Relax. Close your eyes and visualize your arm going around twice as far. Visualize the arm rotating with great ease and going around much further than your first attempt. Visualize the arm easily passing the previous attempt by 30 or 40 degrees. Do this visualization 3 times. After you have done it 3 times open your eyes and make another attempt. You see? Notice how much further your arm has rotated. Visualization works.

There were times when I would sit for long periods of time imagining a healing beam of white light pouring in through my head filling my entire body, especially my legs. I would recollect what it specifically felt like to be strong and fit and become fully associated with these feelings. Not just to think about them but to BECOME THEM.

Meditation helped me to calm my mind and think clearly as well as taught me great discipline to observe the workings of the mind for long periods of time. (If you are interested I suggest Thich Nhat Hanh's book *The Miracle of Mindfulness.*)

I read a lot of books to keep me inspired by the authors mentioned in previous chapters. I got very interested not so much in self-improvement, but in self-transformation. My old self and all of his attitudes, ways of thinking and feeling were the cause of this debilitated state. I didn't want to improve that guy, I wanted to become something new and different altogether. I felt that if I could begin to rewire the workings of my brain and emotions that a different outcome was inevitable. I was quite serious about this idea of transformation.

"Who would I be if I simply dropped all of my present beliefs about myself and the world?" "What kind of a life have these attitudes and beliefs given me up until now?" "Do I really want to continue on in this manner or is it time that I gave up these habits?"

My transformation was in direct proportion to the amount of truth I was willing to hear. I would take a certain idea and think and feel about for days. For instance, Why do you get hurt? Not because of what people do, but because you have demanded that they do as you wish. Abolish all demands, then people can behave any way they like while you remain at peace. I tried to apply these ideas to my struggle and gain new insight and experiences. What if I gave up all demands about how people should behave?

I read Thoreau, Emerson, Plato, Vivekananda, The Tao, Boethius, Hermann Hesse, Marcus Aurelius and many other authors that provided real esoteric teaching and applied it to my life.

I listened to recordings when I wasn't reading. Louise Hay, Carolyn Myss, and Bernie Siegal to name a few, along with Vernon Howard.

I began keeping a journal writing down daily what was going on internally and checking to see that I kept myself in empowered states. Any kind of progress was recorded. I affirmed any and all improvements, not just in my physical state but any significant insight concerning the link between my mind and body. I used this journal to mark my progress, rating my walking ability on a scale of 1 to 10. My first entry was 0.1 the last entry about two years later was 9.8. A "8.0" represented the ability to walk well enough where no one noticed anything wrong with my gait. A "10" represented no debilitation at all.

I paid close attention to the language that I used to speak to others and myself and did my best to use positive language and tones of voice. I realized that we all have tremendous healing capabilities within and I did everything to utilize mine. I had to.

As soon as I accepted my situation (instead of being angry about it) things started to get better. Accepting where I was at, examining how I got there, and beginning to piece together how to eliminate my diseased thinking and feeling put me on the path to recovery. The first noticeable shift was the relaxation of my mind and the lightening of my heart. I was laughing more. I noticed the quality of my sleep improving. I became less fearful and more trusting that everything was exactly as it should be. I read and studied about addictive personalities and how they are formed, and reformed. I listened to uplifting music and did my best to surround myself with positive impressions. Eventually, the body began a slow but progressive journey back to health.

It took close to a year before I could walk with any confidence. I remember the first time I was able to move my big toe. It was a thrill, as it had been months since I had any control over any of my lower limbs. It Really was something to celebrate. I remember just moving the toe over and over again turning the "toe lifting" into sets of repetitions as if I were working out. Which is exactly what was happening. I went from being able to move my toes, to moving my feet, to moving my legs, to standing with the walker, to walking with the walker, to walking with a cane (a very scary progression), to standing without a cane, to walking without a cane.

When I was first able to stand I looked like a feeble 100-year-old man. I could not straighten my legs or my back. With my knees locked by muscle tension in a bent position, I could not support my body weight with my severely atrophied leg muscles and leaned heavily on the walker. I worked every day to straighten and strengthen my legs and back. I would do sets of squats with only a two to three-inch range of motion. As time went on the range of motion increased along with my leg strength.

I set daily goals to achieve in my apartment. "Today I am going to stand for 30 seconds without holding onto the walker, five times." "Today I am going to use my walker to go 25 times back and forth from the kitchen to the bed."

I had a mini-trampoline in my apartment. I ordered an attachment that gave me something to hold on to. I would take my walker over to the trampoline and struggle to step up the four or five inches it took to get on. I would then hold on to the bar and just do a gentle bounce. I had no coordination in my legs but once I got them in position, I was able to do effective movements that immediately increased my circulation, eventually strengthened my entire lower body and the nerve endings that seemed completely dead began to come to life and give some feedback.

There were times that if I didn't know better I would have guessed that two legs were not enough to balance a man. The bottom of my feet felt as if they were round. It seemed absurd that they alone could be used for walking. Of course, intellectually I knew better but it was such a strong feeling of futility and impossibility it is worth mentioning.

Eventually, the day came when I had to give up the walker. The prospect of walking or standing with only a cane was as frightening as standing at the edge of a huge cliff. I was so used to the stability and safety of the walker and had gotten really comfortable using it to get around but that was a comfort I HAD to give up.

It was a VERY difficult transition from the walker to the cane. No more did I have the entire ultra stable mechanism with four legs and a place to grab onto on each side. I noticed I had actually become way too used to the security this device provided. My confidence dropped severely as I stood up with only a cane and I was barely able to balance myself and hardly took a step for the first few days. I would put the cane out in front of me and used my other two legs to form a sort of a tripod. I could balance myself but couldn't really walk. I would just stand there, frightened trying not to fall. I thought it was ridiculous but I promised myself I would NOT go back to the walker. Within a week I was getting around my apartment pretty well with just the cane. I was writing daily reports so I could see I WAS progressing. A month later, I was able to take some steps without the cane.

I started venturing out to the sidewalk. At first taking just a few steps outside my building, which was a big adventure and major achievement. Then walking to the corner. Then crossing the street one day. A frightening experience as it took me five times as long to get across and no matter how much of a head start I had, I couldn't make it across before the light would change. There were a few times I thought I was about to buy it when these cars would come whipping through the New York City intersections after the light had changed and I was still near the middle of the street. It did provide some extra incentive to move quicker than usual.

There were a couple of instances where I would try to hail a cab. They would pull over and when I started walking and wobbling towards the cab, they would speed away, convinced I was drunk. I'm sure I looked like I was drunk, as my legs were so unstable.

I fell hundreds and hundreds of times while learning to stand and walk and did my best to stay light-hearted. There's a saying in boxing "it doesn't matter how many times you go down, it matters how many times you get back up." I kept that in mind. I practiced walking in the basement hallway of my building and the park across the street. I used kneepads and elbow pads to prevent me from getting too banged up.

I actually studied other people walking to try to gain tips from them. I was astonished to notice how much coordination is required for this simple skill we all take for granted. As I watched people walk I noticed that when the feet pass each other the feet are no more than a quarter of an inch apart or less. It's really a very precise movement that we all take for granted. My feet kept banging into each other. The toes of one foot catching the heel of the other was one of the main causes of my falling.

This falling was often difficult to take and I had to struggle not to get too depressed or angry. Here I was literally learning how to walk again, no different than a child, except children don't have all the judgment adults have. Sometimes I ended up in a rage at my condition, how feeble and uncoordinated my legs were. I noticed that my attitude towards falling had a direct impact on my progress. I did my best to stop berating myself or take myself too seriously. I had to go on and the self-damning had to end.

I began to accept that every day I was going to fall . . . a lot. It got to the point where falling stopped being a big deal and I usually had a smile on my face by the time I was on my feet. I stayed relaxed yet very focused on my goals, one of which was to be able to jog two continuous miles one year after I learned to walk again. I made that goal.

While shuffling around my neighborhood I found myself in front of a bike store. The idea of riding a bike again thrilled me as much as scared me. I had not owned a bike for some time. I went in the store and despite being unable to get my leg over the seat, I bought a bike. Now some would say this was a stupid purchase for a man in my condition, but I thought it would give me something to look forward to and to work towards. I stuck my cane in between my backpack and my jacket and walked the bike home holding onto the handlebars. I was thrilled and scared about the prospects.

Today I have regained all of my required-by-life abilities and continue to gain in the athletic arena. I have gone on some extremely challenging hikes in Utah and Maine without difficulty. I ride my bike 5 to 10 miles every day as my mode of transportation in New York City. I am back to weightlifting and yoga. I am able to leg press 500lbs for ten repetitions. I feel as well as I ever have. As far as my athletic abilities go, my physical strength is 100% along with my hand speed and coordination. My legs are a little less coordinated than they used to be, but the feeling and coordination in my hands and fingers have returned completely. I am no longer able to jump or sprint like I used to. I have noticed that I am not required to dunk a basketball or run a sub 5-second 40-yard dash on a daily basis.

If you want to recover

It is necessary to have specific aims or goals, both long term and short term, and to honor those goals by fully committing yourself to making them. Without goals, you are aimless and will be pushed and pulled by your ever-changing nature. How many times have you decided to do something on Monday that was really going to change your life, then you wake up Tuesday morning with absolutely no desire to do what you said you would do? Your goals should be a stretch, something that is going to be hard to achieve and there should be a distinct time frame, daily goals, one-week goals, four-week goals, yearly goals etc. Write your goals down and report on them each day. Make your goals public by telling friends who are in goodwill towards you. That way, you're on the hook to do what you said you would.

It is my belief that all disease is reversible. If you are interested in being healthy, please STUDY HEALTH. Stop giving any credence to medical dogmatism and understand that health is not found in a pill or a bottle or any bizarre toxic treatments. It is impossible to practice health and not get healthier. A common question I get at my lectures is, "Can anybody recover, or are some people too far gone?" I believe that the human spirit combined with the laws of nature are a mighty combination, and when the inner self is transformed the outer self follows suit. How could it possibly hurt for you to believe that you are recovering?

Remember that any difficulty in life can provide an opportunity for growth. We are not here to shrink and cower under our personal difficulties. We are here to grow out of them. A man or a woman's struggle is what makes them who they are. Your illness and wish for health is a chance for immense growth and inner change. See it as the opportunity that it is and find that place in yourself that is willing to face anything.

Ships are safe in the harbor but that is not what ships are for.

Forget the results. Just start your voyage and make the efforts and your life will be richer. Never give up going for what you want. Whether you make it or whether you don't, you'll be the better for your efforts. Good captains do not make their reputation on quiet seas. They make their reputations in severe storms.

Essentials for recovery

Desire and belief

You need 3 strong reasons why you need to get better. Then have a clearly defined goal and a time frame in which to achieve. You need to be quite specific about HOW you will know or measure when you have reached your goal. Write all of this down.

You must not only want to get well you must *believe* you can and begin to ACT AS IF the healing has already begun. Never mind any of the mechanical doubting thoughts and attitudes. Tell them to shut up. You are now too busy healing to listen to them.

A useful affirmation: I AM WELL. Notice not to say I am going to be well or I will be well as that puts the healing in the future. The future is not here. I AM Well. I AM healthy. State your affirmation in the present tense. Say these things out loud and MEAN it. The tone and resonance of your voice are creating a vibration that is felt throughout every cell in your body.

Play with which word you put the emphasis on. "i am WELL." or "i AM well." or "I am well." Or emphasize all three. I AM WELL. Believe what you are giving voice to. Say this and other affirmations as many times a day as you can. Make it a mantra that will begin to burn different pathways and make new connections between the neurons in your brain and your body. Through affirmation, you are imposing your will on the mind and body.

ACT *AS IF*. One of the most powerful tools for transformation. No matter what your ailment, act like you are healthy. Stand or sit in postures of a healthy vibrant person. Speak in tones that evoke confidence and self-assurance. Think the thoughts you would think, feel the emotions you would feel, say the words you would say if healed. Completely take on the character of someone who has a healthy vibrant body now. You may feel strange doing this at first, but as the days and weeks roll on you will have adapted an entirely different way of thinking and feeling. Not only will your mind be different but your body chemistry will have changed.

Take time to close your eyes and visualize your ultimate, healthy self. Make the visualization in color and give it motion. After a while of watching your incredible, healthy self-move around, step into that body and BECOME your healthy self. Feel your strong heartbeat and your powerful body move. Feel the feelings and emotions of a young, healthy, vibrant person. See what you might see in such a state, speak how you might speak and be grateful for what you are experiencing. The more time you can spend in these heightened states the better you will begin to feel. Feeling better is guaranteed and has only to do with how sincere you are in your approach.

If you are saying to yourself "this is silly" and "it won't work for me" you have got to adjust your attitude. If you want to do the impossible, you have to be willing to go to places in yourself that you are extremely uncomfortable with.

Stay inspired. Read stories that uplift and inspire, surround yourself with those you admire. Avoid negativity in all of its forms be it people, movies, magazines, newspapers, television, gossip, etc. Refuse any thought that is not going to aid you in your recovery. AFFIRMING THOUGHTS ONLY. Surround yourself with beauty. LISTEN TO INSPIRING MUSIC.

Stop poisoning the body and do your best to live according to your natural inclinations and diet. You have all the information you need in this book to do so.

Refuse to get involved in ANY negativity, internally or externally. Notice how the body goes into a panic when thinking certain thoughts and STOP IT. Refuse to indulge yourself in ridiculous fantasies that cause you pain and wreak havoc on your body. You know what I am talking about. The pictures and mental movies we all have about a certain event in your life where you did something foolish, mean or hurtful. Or the opposite—how badly someone treated you and running and re-running the event over and over again in your mind. The fantasies of revenge or looking like the hero in front of your friends or co-workers. The horrible practice of imagining the worst possible scenarios in the future and again putting them on repeat in your brain. Know that ALL of this type of thinking is disease producing. If you pay close attention to your body when you are running these mind films, you will actually FEEL how they are harming you. Stop indulging in this harmful practice. Instead, use your imagination to empower yourself.

CLEAN out your living space. You will be amazed what a relief it is to de-clutter your home and rid yourself of all the accumulated, unnecessary stuff in your home. It is a BIG lift to your spirit to live in a clean orderly house.

Be GRATEFUL. Count your blessings at least twice a day. Preferably when you get up in the morning and when you go to sleep. Write down the things that you are grateful for. I don't care how difficult your situation may be, if you're reading this you have something to be grateful for. Your eyes must be working fairly well and you are still breathing. Millions of people did not awaken this morning. You did!!!

Get plenty of fresh air and sunshine. Try to be outside for at least 2 hours every day. Get your bare feet in the grass or at least on the Earth. If you are able to move your body do it and do it consistently and as vigorously as you are able. Minimum 20 minutes of exercising every day.

Limit your time in front of the television and computer. Too much screen time is destructive to the body. Social media is a poor excuse for a social life. Make efforts to actually meet people, in person, face to face. The chances of you experiencing something genuine and life-like will be far greater if you do not stay your computer or phone.

If you can only move certain parts of your body, do it. If you are only able to make certain movements make exercises out of them. For instance: Sit in a chair and lift your arms out to the side, slowly and as high as you can. Bring them back down in a controlled fashion and lift them again. Move the limbs with precision and mindfulness like a dancer. Start by doing 10 repetitions five different times. Rest precisely 1 minute between the sets.

Work up to doing 25 repetitions then put a light weight in your hands and go back to 10 reps. Then work up to 25 reps with the weights. Now do that movement to the front and try to make the same improvements. ANY progress you make will prove immensely beneficial.

Of course, this goes for ANY movement you can do. Any movement you are capable of can become an exercise when done with purpose and mindfulness.

Of course, if you are able-bodied you MUST have a regular exercise regime. Fast walking, biking, weight-training, rebounding (mini-trampoline) tai chi, yoga, swimming etc.

Remember your skin is your number one eliminative organ. Sweating is a great way to detoxify the body.

Any kind of resistance training is great, either weight training and/or calisthenics.

The mini-trampoline or rebounder is an excellent form of exercise that will strengthen your entire body and is a great workout for the heart and lungs. You can use a support bar if you are unsteady on your legs. (The Needak brand rebounders are the best I have seen.)

Not just for your body but for your head and your heart. A good exercise program will increase your confidence, help you to relax, aid your body's eliminative organs, increase your muscle tone, decrease your body fat, increase your heart strength, release endorphins, improve your skin and increase your overall circulation.

If you wish to be healthy you MUST exercise!

Do something creative. Play an instrument, write a story, take an acting class, memorize a great speech, paint a picture. Creativity demands access to other parts of your brain and heart you normally wouldn't be using in your daily life. If you wish to break out of the cycle of dis-ease-producing thoughts and feelings then put yourself in position to have some new and different impressions and access a different part of your brain.

Here are some more suggestions to help turn things around.

- Asking What I Owe vs. Asking What I'm Owed
- Being Grateful vs. Being resentful
- Gaining Understanding vs. Wanting a Quick-fix Solution
- Allowing Solutions vs. Forcing Solutions
- Seeking Contentment vs. Seeking Excitement
- Inwardly Focused vs. Outwardly Focused
- Stubbornness vs. Acceptance
- Do more Listening Less Talking.

12

SUMMARY

Health is not a business.

After reading the first draft of this work an acquaintance asked me, "Why should I listen to you?" "You shouldn't," I told him. "You shouldn't listen to me or be obedient to me or ANY one health professional, nutritionist, association, society unless you know their methods have truly helped others and they have no motive other than to aid you." Take this tremendous opportunity to do one of the rarest things a human being can do . . . THINK FOR YOURSELF. The trouble we could avoid if we were practiced at this rare art of self-reliance and if we would stop assuming that only a credentialed person can have something of value to say and that those without them are not worth a listen. It is a common practice to attack the messenger if the message is not what we expect or want to hear, especially if the message is a threat to business. Assess what you have been presented here, if it seems reasonable, fairly and thoroughly apply the advice to yourself and see if things do not get better. You can have your own empirical evidence, be your own scientist, and work in the most incredible laboratory ever invented, your body.

Concerning "credentials," I have one question for you. Who is in charge of the "health care" system in this country? The answer is the heavily credentialed American Medical Association is in charge. If credentials equal wisdom and competence, why is it that our country in such a dis-ease ridden state and so rapidly on the decline with more obese people than any other country in the world, with more deaths from cancer and heart dis-ease than ever before, and with the most heavily drugged child population mankind has ever known? History has proven time and again that blind faith in our leaders is a disastrous practice.

I hope I have presented you with a logical and sound model for healthy living and a new perspective on dis-ease and health. My wish is that something in you is thinking *this makes sense.* I can assure you that I have personally seen hundreds of sick and dying individuals return themselves to health through these natural means.

You might also want to consider the fact that I am not selling you anything. There are no products to buy, no powders, no special formulas or pills, no new age program, and no way for me to profit from your heeding these suggestions and abiding by Natural Laws.

Any endeavor that grants precious rewards does require great discipline and effort. I am quite aware of what a challenge this new way of living can be (eating according to your biology). I am also conscious of the resistance that may result when you realize the "sacrifices" that you must endure. To some of you, it may seem to be a difficult, if not impossible way of life. You must remember and realize that all of your present habits, good or bad, have been learned and can be unlearned. Do not underestimate what you are capable of doing.

Our brains have been wired, mostly unconsciously, in a certain way to which we have grown accustomed, heavily influenced by our culture, parents, and immediate surroundings. In his book *Your Maximum Mind*, Dr. Herbert Benson of Harvard Medical School describes how this mind organization occurs:

> "Over the years you develop 'circuits' and 'channels' of thought in your brain. These are physical pathways which control the way you think, the way you act, and often the way you feel. Many times these pathways become so fixed, that they turn into what I call 'wiring.' In other words, the circuits or channels become so deeply ingrained that it seems almost impossible to transform them."

There are approximately 100 billion nerve cells in the brain, and each of these communicates with the others through connections called synapses. The total number of possible connections is 25,000,000,000,000, 000,000,000,000,000,000, Dr. Benson estimates. Put another way, if you were to stack sheets of typing paper with each sheet-representing a neuron connection, the resulting pile would be approximately 16 billion light-years high, extending beyond the limits of the known universe.

Robert Ornstein MD, another renowned brain researcher from the University of California, claims that the number of possible connections in the brain is greater than the number of atoms in the universe.

It seems, according to these scientists, that the possibility for our brains making new connections is unlimited. Please do not sell yourself short by thinking that you are your past. You are MUCH greater than you know.

I can only TELL you what a wonderful gift it is to live according to Natural Laws and make you aware of the magnificent benefits this way of life affords me and the growing number of those who are catching on to this wonderful way of life. I can also tell you of the hundreds of people who have been left for dead by today's *health experts* who are now leading disease free vigorous lives with great confidence in their physical abilities without worry that their previous conditions will return. I also can tell you of the guaranteed success of those looking to lose weight, as well as those once afflicted with asthma, diabetes, herpes, "aids," cancer, etc., who are now living drug-free, asymptomatic, healthy lives.

> *The only source of knowledge is experience.*
>
> ≈✶ ALBERT EINSTEIN

You must EXPERIENCE the increased energy, loss of fat, glowing skin, mental alertness, and overall vitality this raw food regimen brings with it in order to UNDERSTAND. It is impossible for you to accurately imagine the benefits, and to try to do so is a big mistake.

The idea that you will be living a life of deprivation is an illusion equivalent to telling a prisoner he should stay in his rat-infested jail cell because he will miss the wildlife if he were to walk out. Eventually, you will not be missing anything and you will be thrilled with your new way of life. It may take some time, but if you make sincere efforts towards this transition, the rewards to be experienced are beyond your imagination.

As far as the idea of deprivation and being bored by the natural regime, I can assure you that there is simply no serious raw-foodists complaining of boredom. After a while, your body will re-establish its natural cravings. This transition to health may take a year or two. It makes sense to consider the time your body has spent on the normal toxic diet and to realize that weaning yourself off the addictive foods and additives requires some work. Those who have made a sincere and lasting effort have nothing but praise and stories of delightful transformation. I can remember on many occasions complaining that there was "nothing to eat" when I was on the S.A.D. diet. Of course being bored about what to eat has nothing to do with lack of food choices, it is simply indicative of the deranged attitude we have towards food.

Comfort foods are the foods that make you the most uncomfortable.

Eating with the idea of entertaining ourselves creates food addiction and will lead to an unending passionate quest that can never be satisfied.

It is quite an experience to taste a fruit the way it was meant to be tasted with re-awakened, re-sensitized taste buds. It is a whole other sense of wonder to have your body operating the way in which it was intended, with improved digestion, vision, and hearing, something very few human beings ever experience. Making the transition may be a challenge, but I assure you there is nothing boring about living according to your true nature, in fact, it may be the most exciting thing you have ever experienced. Making this transition is the equivalent of running your car in first gear for years and all of a sudden discovering that there are three other gears.

You will also save a considerable amount of money by staying healthy, avoiding regular trips to the doctor, and having no need to buy any type of remedial product, prescription, or over-the-counter drugs. If you or a family member becomes ill, there will be no question of how to deal with it. It is also important to realize that there is an entire world of raw food preparation available to you. There are many raw food preparation books on the market these days. I am pleased to see that the idea of raw eating is catching on.

Excessive care of the body, is most inimical to the practice of virtue.

≡✷ PLATO

Unfortunately, many of these preparation manuals have included heavily spiced, processed and irritating menus. It would be best to avoid using molasses, refined sugars, onions, garlic, table or sea salt, pepper, and any processed food or liquid.

If you are seriously ill or have been suffering from chronic health problems for years, a resolute and stringent discipline may be required for your recovery. An immediate and complete cessation of any foods and toxins that do not belong to the body and an adherence to Natural Laws may make the difference between life and death. In such cases, strict compliance with proper feeding and care of the body is paramount.

If you are not in such a debilitated physical condition, it would behoove you to recognize the difficulty of the task at hand and to take a reasonable approach to making this life-changing transition. There are some people that come upon this knowledge and immediately take it upon themselves to give up all their unnatural feeding habits. This type of complete and determined effort is rare under normal circumstances. Assessing and measuring the difficulties you may incur is a wise move, especially when there are others in your household. Way too often families are disrupted and irreparably upset because of a reformed individual that insists, "everyone must change now that I have." This is a sort of violence that can be more dis-ease producing than a drug-laden steak.

Remember that eating right is a major factor in, the quality of our health, but it is not the most important one. It may be more important to keep the peace in your home rather than fighting to change everybody now that you're ready to change. I suggest if these ideas of living resonate in you and you have the interest and inclination to begin to live according to Nature's Laws. Do it for yourself at first without imposing your will on any friends or family. There is nothing more inviting than the power of example. It is possible that others will also see the benefits of this way of life.

Certainly, you can present these ideas to your family members and loved ones. You can SUGGEST that they read this book. If they are resistant, do yourself and them a favor and LEAVE THEM ALONE.

Do not try to change others.

It is extremely frustrating to see family members and loved ones involved in daily poisoning acts and thoughtless, ravaging "treatments" that you know are absurd and dangerous. However, it is equally absurd to try to change somebody who does not want to change. One of the most difficult lessons I have learned and continue to learn is that some people would rather die horrible deaths than change. This is a fact that is sometimes hard to swallow but is clearly evident throughout our society. There is not one adult in the civilized world that does not know that smoking causes cancer and death, yet millions of people continue to engage in this activity and spend their money to kill themselves.

I once saw a man who, after thirty years of smoking, had to have major throat surgery for the cancer that had invaded his esophagus and vocal cords. After the operation, he had to be fed through a plastic tube inserted in his neck.

Now devoid of vocal chords and a large part of his neck, unable to speak or eat, this man insisted on his smoking pleasure and would put a lit cigarette into the tube and inhale. This is a testimony to the willfulness and obdurate nature of human beings disinterested in change.

Just because what you are proposing is tried, tested, true, and effective, not everybody wants to hear it. In fact, MOST people do not want to hear it. Some of the greatest teachers ever to walk this planet were mocked, ostracized, persecuted, and put to death because of the truthful message they imparted. Do not waste your energy trying to force a change in others.

Remember the fact that we live in an insane world. Any moves or efforts towards sanity will absolutely guarantee accusations and charges of insanity from the insane.

Do not put yourself in harm's way by making an issue of your new way of living. Most people do not want to hear it, and you are doing yourself damage by bringing it up to the disinterested.

Obsessive behavior

Most people do not take any time to examine their eating habits or consider the consequences of just eating like everybody else. Obviously, there is a price to pay for this lack of responsibility. On the other end of the spectrum, there are those who become obsessive about their eating choices and unreasonable when it comes to their physical maintenance. This type of compulsion and rigid neurotic behavior is dis-ease producing in and of itself and makes for a very unpleasant person.

Enthusiasm and excitement are imminent as you learn about and experience the effects of eating well and caring for the body. I certainly encourage you to share your joy and enthusiasm with those who are interested.

Unfortunately, there are those who will take the idea of nutrition WAY too far and make it the only focus in their life.

Balance is lost by obsessive and exaggerated attention devoted to nutrition. It is one thing to be dedicated and disciplined about the care of your body, it is another thing to be overly concerned and neurotic about it. A life unbalanced is painful and dis-ease producing.

My suggestion is that you assess your personal condition and your lifestyle, consider exactly what you would like to achieve in terms of improving your health, make some specific goals, do your best to achieve them, and let go of the result. However, if you are in physical pain and/or gravely ill I suggest an intense level of commitment. Do not forget to keep a sense of humor about yourself and enjoy the process.

There are those who use their eating habits as a means to express their anger, avoid others, feel superior, and distract themselves from the real issues in their lives by compulsively talking and thinking about eating. I highly suggest you avoid this type of behavior. If you find yourself constantly defending yourself and arguing with others, you can bet that you are doing more harm than good. It is fairly easy to tell who is interested in these ideas and who is not. Learn to

> *"Truth is our element of life, yet if a man fasten his attention on a single aspect of truth and apply himself to that alone for a long time, the truth becomes distorted and not itself but falsehood."*
>
> ➤ EMERSON

be diplomatic and to disengage those that want to argue and fight and relish those who have a sincere interest in improving their health.

Remember that there is nothing more important to your well being than the contents of your heart and mind. If you are constantly tense, anxiety-ridden, angry, resentful, and worried, your chances of achieving health are negligible.

We are spiritual beings in a physical body, act accordingly and feed your spirit. Starting your day with a sitting meditation is a most beneficial practice. Do something creative on a daily basis, something you love. Challenge yourself to go outside your comfort zones. Learn to sing, paint, draw or dance. It really doesn't matter what you pick what matters is that you use your brain and body in new and challenging ways. Keeping a daily journal will allow your mind to slow down, give you the ability to assess just what it is that may be bothering you, and give you a clear opportunity to express yourself. Reading the works of great minds, many whom have been quoted in this book, will provide you with constant inspiration to reach above and beyond the daily quagmire of mechanical thinking and unconscious behavior so prevalent in today's world. Of course, eating properly will be a tremendous aid to your spiritual growth, as a finely tuned body increases one's receptivity to higher ideas.

Exercise is essential to our well being, and going without a regular physical regime is harmful to your body. A gentle discipline is necessary. Do not count activity such as walking to work or cleaning the house as exercise. Spend at least fifteen to twenty minutes a day doing some type of disciplined exercise where there is no distraction. Weight training, calisthenics, swimming (find a pool without chlorine) and fast walking are all very effective disciplines. If you do not have any equipment or resources you can get in great shape using calisthenics (see my video on YouTube: "Full Body Workout, No equipment" on "Health Tips With Matthew Grace"[1]). Wherever there is a floor you can train. Do not waste your energy making excuses why you cannot exercise. If you do not have twenty minutes a day to spend on yourself, your lifestyle must change.

Make sure you leave some time, even if it is only a half an hour a week (although I do suggest more), to do some kind of activity that you enjoy, such as playing a musical instrument, sculpting, dancing, singing, painting, or drawing. These artistic endeavors can also be a tremendous boon to your well being.

One of the most common situations I come across when counseling sickly individuals is their tendency to make themselves SO busy that they have "legitimate" excuses for not taking proper care of themselves. Staying busy is a disease in and of itself that is sure to manifest itself physically. The desperation to constantly be on the run or on the phone or DOING something is evidence of great emotional turmoil that is being ignored and, even worse, denied. Most of the world is doing this in some form or another, and this staying overly busy is the cause of great physical, mental, and emotional anguish. We

---

1   Available on YouTube: https://youtu.be/4ipQyhpZR8U

are human beings, not human doings. Most people are frightened of a quiet moment because that would mean facing themselves. Therefore, we have invented endless arrays of distractions to take the attention off what really needs attention. Eating is a prime distraction, along with texting, tweeting, over-working, smoking, drinking, television, talking, focusing on others, creating or involving ourselves in some type of human conflict or emergency.

Our problems gain size and strength with each evasion. The more we run from our problems, the more they show up in our lives. The more they show up in our lives, the more we need to distract ourselves . . . a truly vicious cycle. The opposite is thankfully true. If you are willing to stand and face the difficulties in your life, those difficulties will LOSE power and strength, and YOU will gain power and strength. Then you will no longer be a constant slave to your obsessive behaviors and avoidances, and gain some balance in your life. The "freedom" that most people talk about is an insatiable never-ending sensual slavery. The only true freedom that exists lies in an obedience to higher laws.

Living in the dark is dangerous.

Just because most of the world is living in the dark and you have grown accustomed to the world's habitual pains and sufferings do not mean you must go on smashing into the furniture or falling down and injuring yourself. There is A WAY OUT. You have a choice. Every second you are choosing whether to think in your old familiar ways or to try something different. If you do what you have always done, you get what you have always gotten. A good definition of insanity is doing the same thing but expecting a different result. Allowing yourself to be formed and molded by a society gone mad is a guarantee that YOU will also be mad.

If these ideas make sense to you and you wish to implement this program, I would suggest that you make a consistent and regular study of this book. It is one thing to read this once and think it makes sense, it is another thing to summon up the necessary energy and desire to go against years of mis-education and indoctrination. Do not underestimate the force of belief. The ideas in this book are a tremendous threat to the status quo, and implementing these ideas requires great confidence and constant reenforcement of these ideas.

Making these conscious choices to change your eating habits is a sign that you no longer want to live the way most people do. You are affirming that you will no longer succumb to your addictive and destructive behaviors in the physical world. These efforts, combined with the reawakening of the body, increase the receptivity of your being which allows for a greater possibility for inner transformation and your overall wellness.

Good luck. Have fun.

Believe me, it is great fun to KNOW how to stay Healthy and keep yourself and your family away from the madness of "modern medicine" and their dangerous drugging regimes and surgeries. It is incredibly freeing to UNDERSTAND

Health and realize that you are in control of your well being and "luck" has nothing to do with it. It is a wonderful thing to be free of the fear that you may get a serious disease that "cannot be cured." It is also a lot of fun to look and feel years younger than you actually are and be a living example of Health! It is also a wonderful thing to be your own doctor and your own family doctor. It is also a wonderful thing to live in a healthy, fit, well functioning body with no addictions or dependence on any drugs.

I am certain the day will come when people will look back at our present-day society and wince at the fact that doctors prescribed KNOWN POISONS as "treatments" for their patients and that their patients were too brainwashed to see the danger and absurdity of this practice. Our modern-day society and "health experts" are amused at many of the archaic, medieval treatments such as bloodletting and the applying of leeches to the skin of sick patients that was once practiced by "trusted" physicians, yet these days they see no problem with injecting their patient's veins with mustard gas ("chemotherapy") or injecting mercury into babies (vaccines) to supposedly increase their chances of being healthy.

If you or a loved one have been told that you are doomed to live with "incurable" or "chronic" disease, you have been lied to. You do not have to suffer through the druggings, burnings, poisonings, mutilations, irradiations, and hopelessness prescribed to you. You now have the opportunity to do what thousands of others have done, you can take responsibility for your well being, understand the true nature of dis-ease, the simplicity of health and allow your body to do what it knows best—heal.

ABOUT THE AUTHOR

Matthew Grace was diagnosed with "incurable disease." He was unable to stand or move his legs. Gripped by severe numbness and fatigue, he was paralyzed and given little hope for any recovery and no chance to walk again. Refusing ALL conventional treatments and working from the inside out, this man, doomed by modern medicine, found his way back to health, strength, and vitality.

A former standout boxer, fitness expert, health advocate, public speaker and author, his services as a trainer and health consultant have been sought out by people all over the world, including many celebrities. The President and Founder of the Coalition for Health Re-education, Grace has helped thousands of people regain their health.

He has appeared on ABC's Prime Time Live, Good Day New York on Fox News and has been interviewed on many national radio programs. He was the host of a cable program in New York City for more than 7 years and for more than 20 years he has been inspiring audiences with his remarkable story. His mission "to let people know there is A Way Out, no matter what health challenge you may be facing," is complemented by his insightful, philosophical and often humorous delivery.

www.matthewgrace.com

DISCLAIMER

Matthew Grace is not a medical doctor and does not prescribe medicine or treatments for disease. This book is a study of The Laws of Nature and is written to re-mind the reader that Health is a birthright, simple and attainable by all.

CPSIA information can be obtained
at www.ICGtesting.com
Printed in the USA
FFHW020509271018
48942723-53183FF